Reflections on the Challenges of Psychiatry in the UK and Beyond

A psychiatrist's chronicle from
deinstitutionalisation to community care

Nick Bouras

Pavilion

Reflections on the Challenges of Psychiatry in the UK and Beyond

A psychiatrist's chronicle from deinstitutionalisation to community care

© Nick Bouras 2017

Published by:
Pavilion Publishing and Media Ltd
Rayford House, School Road, Hove, East Sussex, BN3 5HX
Tel: 01273 434 943
Fax: 01273 227 308
Email: info@pavpub.com

Published 2017

ISBN: 978-1-911028-41-3

Author: Nick Bouras
Production editor: Ruth Chalmers, Pavilion Publishing and Media Ltd
Cover design: Tony Pitt, Pavilion Publishing and Media Ltd
Page layout and typesetting: Emma Dawe, Pavilion Publishing and Media Ltd
Printing: CPI Anthony Rowe

Contents

About the author

Nick Bouras MD, PhD, FRCPsych, is professor emeritus of psychiatry at the Institute of Psychiatry, King's College London and honorary consultant psychiatrist at South London and the Maudsley Foundation NHS Trust. He is currently programme director of Maudsley International.

Professor Bouras led the research programme of the first Community Mental Health Centre in the UK and carried out extensive studies of service monitoring evaluation. He was consultant psychiatrist at Guy's Hospital of South London and the Maudsley Foundation NHS Trust for over 25 years and was instrumental in the re-provision of services from three large psychiatric institutions. Professor Bouras participated actively in the development of community-based multi-professional mental health services that have been supporting numerous residential facilities in local communities for people with intellectual disabilities and complex mental health needs, people with chronic schizophrenia, and other neurodevelopmental disorders.

Professor Bouras initiated the development of the Estia (Evaluation, Services, Training, Intervention, Assessment) Centre, (www.estiacentre.org) and remained director until his retirement. This was and remains an innovative concept combining clinical services, training and research & development, jointly funded by the NHS and University. His research has been focused on health service related topics including assessment and clinical effectiveness of specialist mental health services, evaluation of multi-professional training methods, and social and biological determinants of behaviour in psychiatric patients.

Reflections on the Challenges of Psychiatry in the UK and Beyond
© Pavilion Publishing and Media Ltd and its licensors 2017.

«Μη εν πολλοίς ολίγα λέγε, αλλά εν ολίγοις πολλά»

Pythagoras, 6th century BC
'Do not say a little in many words, but a great deal
in a few'

This book is dedicated to the memory of Jim Watson.

Foreword

The article 'Psychiatry in jeopardy' was published by Kenneth Rawnsley in 1984.[1] It is about the fundamental ambivalence within societies, and evident in individuals, towards the substance of psychiatry. Perhaps, in part at least, this derives from a fascination with and anxiety about madness, sex and death, three of the major themes that our speciality has to deal with every day. Rawnsley's article mentions issues that are prominent in Professor Nick Bouras' account in this book. For example, concerns were already widespread about the role, or even need for, a psychiatrist in the field of mental handicap; it was hoped that changing the name of the subject, this time from mental handicap to learning difficulties, then to learning disabilities and currently to intellectual disabilities, might help reduce the social stigma affecting people with this condition.

Professor Nick Bouras has given an account of a career devoted to navigating through the sea of anti-psychiatric biases, while dealing with policies often fuelled by doctrinaire prejudice, bedevilled by management changes and sometimes incompetence, and sometimes dominated by often unfortunate financial preoccupations and complexities. Therefore, Professor Nick Bouras' book could be read with relevance by anyone interested in the past, present and above all future of the NHS, particularly with respect to one of the most disadvantaged groups of all: people with mental handicap (using old terminology for the moment).

---

1   Rawnsley K (1984) Psychiatry in jeopardy. *British Journal of Psychiatry* **145** (6) 573–578.

It seems to me that a rational basis for the services that should be provided for people with mental handicap can be set out in relation to the plans for the closure of Darenth Park Hospital, and their implementation, detailed in this account (see also Chapter 5). This rational basis would begin with the principle that everyone currently in a hospital should be in the location that is best for them. If it turned out that none of the residents of the hospital needed to be there and all could be moved elsewhere, then the hospital could close. The first rational step to implement this with respect to Darenth Park would be to assess the needs of all the residents. This is what was done. Equally rational was the division, on the basis of their assessed needs, of the residents into groups with low (the most numerous group), medium and high (the smallest group) levels of need. Particular attention was paid to the numbers of staff who would be needed to care for the individuals in the setting most suitable for them.

Also rational was the decision to begin by making plans for the most numerous group, those with the lowest levels of need. Despite some difficulties, this entire group was resettled in houses in the community. The mid-need group needed more staff and progress towards resettlement was slower. By the time the focus moved to the most disabled group, it was time for those responsible for finance to review expenditure. They recommended that staff costs were far too high. It was conveniently forgotten that staff requirements had been calculated after needs had been assessed. This exemplifies the practice, unhappily widespread in the NHS generally and perhaps in the mental health services in particular, for financial considerations to prevail over clinical ones. Much time and energy was spent by Professor Nick Bouras and (far too many) others in trying to mitigate the pernicious effects of this practice.

Everyone would agree, I think, that people with a wide range of skills are needed to provide a comprehensive service for a (any) group of patients (or clients). So teams are essential. There is no straightforward way of mapping required skills on to membership of any (or no) professional group. Nevertheless, this does not excuse the interprofessional squabbles and power struggles, let alone ideological claptrap, that have bedevilled mental health service development – and perhaps particularly mental handicap service development – during the past several decades. Running a successful team requires, in my view, only adherence to two basic principles: the 'limit of competence' and the 'network'. This means that every team member must be aware of their own personal limits and the identity of the network, so that in particular circumstances they can say, 'I don't know what to do, but there is someone in the team who does, and I know who they are and can contact them at once.'

In principle, the role definitions of team members should not present difficulty. In reality, however, problems derived from ideological, professional and social power concerns, much of it anti-psychiatric, have made the process anything but straightforward. This a sorry tale, documented in a sober way in these pages. It is most evident in the matter of the role of the psychiatrist in mental handicap, and the need for inpatient residential provision – already noted by Kenneth Rawnsley so long ago. Societal ambivalence about these two issues has also been evident within psychiatry, including within the Royal College of Psychiatrists.

It seems to me that psychiatry has not always been helpful to itself in this, by failing to be crystal clear about how to define the limits of the population properly covered by the term mental handicap (now 'intellectual disabilities'). There was a time when categories of moderate and severe mental handicap were defined in terms of IQ measurement. Whatever one thinks of this practice, it did potentially give guidance as to the size of the problem, with obvious implications for needs for staff, services and, above all, money. This is because of the statistics of IQ measurement: the average IQ is set at 100, with standard deviation 15. (In reality, intelligence is not exactly normally distributed, but this does not affect this point.) Limiting the speciality to below IQ 30 points would cover at most five per cent of the population, while with an upper limit of 70 more than a quarter would be included – an enormous difference. In fact, eschewing IQ as a measure of intellectual disability (ID) has not led to a satisfactory replacement definition of the condition, leading, in my view, to a conceptual muddle that has conflated psychiatric illness, disturbed behaviour, with resulting substantial overlap between ID and generic services. Much of this is documented in what follows. It would have been much better if most of this disputatious story had not needed to be written.

Nevertheless, it is vital to remember that how civilised a society is can be assessed by finding out how it cares for, in particular, people with ID and elderly people with dementia, two groups whose care cannot *par excellence* be justified on the economic grounds now all-pervasive in society.

Another principle illustrated by Professor Nick Bouras' account is that sober scientific and academic input can and should inform service planning and delivery. These pages mention many examples where data collection assisted, or should have assisted, the development of improved services. Sometimes the data went counter to the prevailing policy and the ideology that powered it. I recall an animated discussion of a data set concerning the early work of the Lewisham Mental Health Advice Centre (see also Chapter 2), which was established with the aim of reducing pressure on inpatient admission. In fact, not only did admissions increase, but the total number of people seen increased substantially, due to the easier availability of help for people with previously unmet need.

It turns out that Professor Nick Bouras has had exactly the right mix of personal and professional qualities required for successful work in this difficult field during this period of time. His capacity for working with colleagues from every kind of background is extraordinary; and I am amazed that he has retained details of meetings, documents and personnel as evidenced here. It has been a personal pleasure to have him as a colleague in my department and, particularly in the early days, to work closely with him. His doctoral work concerned with inpatients complemented my own,[2,3] and our joint chapter on the nature of the ward environment could (says he modestly) be studied with advantage by those involved with the residents of community facilities as well as hospitals.[4]

James Watson, MD, FRCP, FRCPsych*
Emeritus Professor of Psychiatry, Guy's and St Thomas' Hospitals

*While this book was in production James (Jim) Watson sadly passed away.

---

2   Bouras N (1979) *The Disturbed Behaviour of Patients in Psychiatric Wards* [PhD thesis]. University of London.

3   Watson JP (1974) *Illness and Milieu: A Study of Psychiatric Patients in Hospital* [MD thesis]. University of Cambridge.

4   Watson JP & Bouras N (1988) Psychiatric ward environments and their effects on patients. In: K GranvilleGrossman (Ed.) *Recent Advances in Psychiatry* (pp135–160). London: Churchill Livingston.

Introduction

This book is a personal journey though British psychiatry, the NHS and academic life since 1974, when I arrived in Oxford from Greece, until 2008, the time of my retirement. It describes my experiences as perceived by a postgraduate student, practising clinician, teacher, trainer, researcher and health service manager. It is a personal testament of events witnessed over time, reflecting my own views and involvement in a variety of events.

I joined British psychiatry at a time when it seemed a golden age full of optimism and the excitement of new ideas, plans and proposals. I witnessed major ideological trends in mental health and psychiatry, such as deinstitutionalisation, community care, normalisation theory, advocacy and empowerment. In fact, I participated in the implementation of most of these as an active player in clinical, academic and management positions. Service users and families had great benefits from these trends and changes, and for the majority of them they resulted in a better quality of life. There were, however, problems, particularly for certain groups of service users. My interest was focused initially in service developments for adults with mental illness, and then for people with intellectual disabilities and mental health problems.

The aim of writing this book is to present a personal historical chronicle and a panoramic view of some of the significant events of modern psychiatry as

seen and experienced by a practising psychiatrist
with a diverse background. The book does not refer
to actions or possible other significant events that
might have occurred during this period of which
I did not have personal involvement. The process of
developing mental health services through a maze
of policies, sometimes contradictory, but also with
strong ideological, sociological and political contents,
proved to be very challenging. I also want to show my
appreciation and admiration for the NHS, with its
unique characteristics of universal cover and access
at the point of contact for everyone, including those
with mental health problems. In addition, I hope that
the outstanding contribution of the NHS to training
and research and development (R&D) will emerge
throughout the book, and the added value of strong
links with university academic departments will
be evident.

A significant part of this book concerns the
development of specialist services for people with
intellectual disabilities and mental health problems,
including the controversies surrounding this area.
Successes and disappointments are also featured
throughout. The book is based on personal archives and
notes kept over time, as well as on discussions with
colleagues with whom I had been working closely over
the years.

One of the main problems I faced was the ongoing
changing terminology used to describe conditions as
well as organisations and concepts. When I first started
working in the field, the term mental handicap was
used in the UK and mental retardation in the US.
Then the term changed to learning difficulties and
then to learning disabilities in the UK, while in the
USA and the rest of the world it became developmental
disabilities and then intellectual disabilities. The phrase

Reflections on the Challenges of Psychiatry in the UK and Beyond
© Pavilion Publishing and Media Ltd and its licensors 2017.

intellectual disabilities has also been adopted in the UK, while the new classification systems are likely to introduce new terms such as intellectual developmental disorder. In this book I have kept the terms as they originally appeared in documents and written accounts, and have used intellectual disabilities in most other circumstances. Unavoidably, in certain parts of the book all the terms will appear together, but the meaning will be the same whether the text refers to mental handicap, mental retardation, learning disabilities or intellectual disabilities. Several people are mentioned throughout the book with whom I had professional encounters, and some of them are referred to more than once as we worked together on a number of projects and at various times over the years. References are not included in the book but occasional footnotes referring to publications and other points may be helpful for the reader.

I would like to mention the key people with whom I undertook most of the ventures described in this book and to whom I am most grateful. The late Professor Jim Watson, Dr Raghu Gaind and Dr Maurice Lipsedge have been a constant source of support during their time as consultant psychiatrists at Guy's Hospital. Dr Jed Boardman and Professor Tom Craig have been close colleagues for many years. Dr David Brooks was my first junior doctor in training and remained a close colleague. Dr Geraldine Holt was my first senior registrar and then consultant colleague with whom I undertook many ventures in services, training and research. I am really indebted to her for all her assistance. Mei Jones played a decisive role in the development of the services and shaped up the most crucial role of the community psychiatric nurse (CPN). Lynette Kennedy took over from Mei and has offered us the most skilful team leadership. Steve Hardy was an excellent colleague and gave his consistent support to the training developments of the Estia Centre; he has my gratitude. I am also grateful to Professor Graham Thornicroft for his support at the Institute of Psychiatry. Peter Reading and Stuart Bell were most supportive of our plans, and Mark Allen was an enabling service director with a fine perception of service needs.

Over the years I have also been very fortunate and honoured to enjoy the support and friendship of esteemed colleagues with whom I have not had a direct working collaboration: Dr Jim Birley, Professor John Cox and Dr Douglas Bennett.

Chris Laming and Jenny Martin have given invaluable administrative support.

I am also indebted for their comments on early drafts of this book to Professor German Berrios, Professor Edgar Jones, Professor Tom Craig, Tracey Power, Jim Power, Dr Jean O'Hara, Dr Colin Hemmings and Dr Jane McCarthy. I also express my gratitude to Ruth Chalmers and Jan Alcoe of Pavilion Publishing and Media for their outstanding cooperation and excellent quality of services.

Finally I would like to thank my family and especially my wife Maria for her patience and support and my daughters and Christine and Irene who were deprived of many outings while I had to stay in drafting and writing multiple documents and articles.

The personal notes and archives used as the basis for writing this book, together with those kept from professional life at Guy's Hospital and the Institute of Psychiatry, which fills 62 boxes, have been donated to the Archives Department of King's College London. I'm grateful to Kate O'Brien for accepting them.

Chapter 1: Early years

Arrival

I arrived in Oxford from Greece with my wife Maria at the end of January 1974 to pursue postgraduate training in psychiatry. My wife, being a qualified architect, registered at the London School of Economics for an MSc in town planning, an area that was very popular among young architects in Greece. We both intended to return to Greece as soon as we had achieved our postgraduate aims.

I had completed my training in psychiatry at the Eginition University Hospital of Athens University Medical School and I was a qualified psychiatrist in Greece, having done one year in general medicine, one year in neurology and one year in psychiatry. In addition, I had some primary care clinical experience from my military service with the Hellenic Air Force and the compulsory medical service in the province of Patras District General Hospital. The chairman of the Department of Psychiatry in Athens where I trained was the then newly appointed Professor Costas Stefanis, who later became well known internationally as president of the World Psychiatric Association (WPA) from 1983 to 1990. At that time there was a major issue with Soviet Union dissidents and the main Soviet Union

Psychiatric Association had been expelled from the WPA. Professor Stefanis had a strong background in neurophysiology and was educated mostly in Canada and the USA. Soon after his appointment as chairman of the Psychiatric University Department, he brought in as senior lecturers three British-educated psychiatrists: Aris Liakos, trained at the department of psychiatry at St George's Hospital Medical School under Professor Arthur Crisp; George Christodoulou, trained at the Bethlem and Maudsley Hospital under Dr Denis Leigh; and John Boulougouris, trained at the Maudsley Hospital under Professor Isaac Marks. I was directly accountable as trainee to John Boulougouris whose senior lecturer was Andreas Rambavilas, also British-educated. So my psychiatric training in the middle of the 1970s had been considerably influenced by the orientation of British psychiatry. My mentors Boulougouris and Rambavilas had persuaded me not to seek a scholarship and join the clinical assistant scheme at the Maudsley, but to seek a junior post in order to gain some real clinical experience from psychiatric practice in Britain. My ultimate aim was to obtain a research degree, which was necessary if I was to follow an academic career on my return to Greece.

I applied and was accepted as senior house officer at St John's Hospital in Stone near Aylesbury. It was a medium-sized mental hospital with a good reputation, near Oxford and not far from London. St John's was surrounded by green valleys and blossoming trees, which at springtime created an idyllic picture of the English countryside. We were offered hospital accommodation in a comfortable semi-detached house opposite the hospital grounds, and I started working straight away. I was assigned to an acute admission ward with Dr Charles Bagg as consultant, a very pleasant English child psychiatrist with a classical education who was proud to quote ancient Greek from time to time! He had the busiest catchment area and acute admissions ward. The rule at that time was that I had to complete up to one month of 'clinical attachment' and then be recommended to the General Medical Council for 'temporary registration'. I was approved for temporary registration within two weeks and was offered a contract as senior house officer at St John's Hospital. Having trained in Greece, I did not find the clinical work difficult and was able to take a history, make a diagnosis and recommend treatment. It took me, however, some time to adjust to the service system, particularly the interaction with GPs and the police, and the requirements of the Mental Health Act. When I was on call I had to make decisions on my own, deciding, in particular, whether to admit someone or not, and that was difficult. This was more complicated if there were no vacant beds, which was not uncommon even at that time, or if the police brought in people with alcohol or substance misuse issues in the middle of the night, whom they had found wandering in the nearby towns.

These were new experiences for me, as practising psychiatry at that time in Greece was very different from in England. Greek psychiatry was slowly coming out from a psychoanalytic orientation to a biopsychosocial approach but was predominately asylum-based. There were two overcrowded long-stay psychiatric hospitals at the outskirts of Athens and another one for people with ID. There was still use of unmodified electroshock therapy (ECT) and psychiatrists used to wear a white coat – which was not the case in England! In addition to the acute admission ward at St John's, I was also responsible for two long-stay old age wards with dementia patients. I was amazed to find out that these were known as 'Polish wards', as they held patients of Polish origin who had fought with Britain during the Second World War. St John's Hospital had several acute admissions wards, long-stay wards, a small psychology department mostly carrying out psychometric tests, occupational therapy and social work departments, and outpatient clinics in the nearby district general hospitals. Our outpatient clinic was at the High Wycombe District General Hospital, and an inpatient unit and a day hospital there were also affiliated with St John's[5]. The medical director at St John's Hospital was Dr David Watt, a very gentle, caring and fatherly figure who had been a psychiatrist at Maudsley and had a regular stream of Australian trainees hoping to pass the membership exam of the Royal College of Psychiatrists. There was also at St John's a small research department, and Dr Ian Falloon was a senior registrar conducting a clinical trial with the, at that time, new antipsychotic medication pimozide. Ian Falloon later became well known for his research with families of patients with schizophrenia. St John's Hospital was well organised and ran smoothly with caring nursing staff. Within three months of being at St John's I felt confident in my work and was promoted to a registrar post.

I soon recognised, however, that my main objective of obtaining a higher postgraduate degree and then progressing my academic career in Greece was not going to be realised at St John's. This belief was further fuelled by my friend Christos Paschalis, a Greek psychiatrist doing his PhD in Sheffield with Professor Alec Jenner. Christos insisted that I had to move on soon to an academic department of psychiatry. I discussed this issue with my consultants at St John's who recommended that I first pass the membership exam of the Royal College

5   Crammer J (1990) *Asylum History: Buckinghamshire County Pauper Lunatic Asylum – St John's*. London: Gaskell.

of Psychiatrists and then seek a research position. The membership exam had no value for me in Greece because I had already obtained there the equivalent qualification before coming to Britain. What I needed was a PhD degree, which would have be equivalent to a doctorate recognised in Greece. I was reluctant to start the process of an exam that would have been of no use for my academic career in Greece. I was an uncommon case and the senior colleagues at St John's were very supportive of my wish to fulfil my career aims but also wanted me to continue working there. Dr David Watt arranged for me to obtain clinical experience in the Highfield Adolescent Unit at Warnford Hospital in Oxford, one of the very few such units in England at that time, with Consultant Child Psychiatrist Dr William Parry-Jones, who later became professor of child and adolescent mental health at Glasgow University Medical School. In addition, I attended the Department of Child Psychiatry at Great Ormond Street Hospital with Professor Philip Graham, who had one of best-organised and most academically stimulating departments. I also met Professor Michael Gelder, newly elected professor of psychiatry at Oxford who felt that doing a PhD at Oxford would have been difficult, particularly as he had just taken up his professorial post.

In June 1974 I took my first two weeks' annual leave and went back to Greece for a holiday. Greece was still under dictatorship, and on the day we were to return to Britain the Turkish invaded Cyprus. I was called up by the military and unable to travel back to the UK. It was a very unpleasant and rather frightening experience. I had to stay on an air base in the Peloponnese for a week, with the prospect of going to an active war zone. As soon as I was released I went to Athens Airport with my wife and British Airways put us on the first flight back to London, allowing us to return to St John's. While

Cyprus suffered a major tragedy, with part of its territory being occupied by the Turkish army, the junta regime in Greece collapsed and the country returned to democracy. A climate of euphoria prevailed in the country, which was full of optimism for the future, and this encouraged me to accelerate my efforts to find a PhD position and return to Greece after completing my PhD.

Guy's Hospital

In the meantime, my mentor from Greece, John Boulougouris, recommended me to Professor Jim Watson, who had just been appointed professor of psychiatry at Guy's Hospital Medical School. Jim Watson interviewed me and accepted me as a PhD student on condition that for the two-year registration period I funded myself. I was successful in securing private funding from Greece, and in October 1975 I left St John's for Guy's Hospital in London. That was the start of a collaboration with Jim Watson that lasted for 35 years – and which features frequently throughout this book. The academic Department of Psychiatry at Guy's was small at that time, and in addition to Jim Watson there were Bernie Rosen as senior registrar in psychiatry and Tom Trauer as clinical psychologist. Both came to Guy's, together with Jim Watson, from the department of psychiatry of St George's Hospital Medical School. I was based in the basement of the building at 10 Newcomen Street, together with another PhD student, Dr Salem Rabee, a psychiatrist from Iraq. Jenny Wilson-Barnet also joined us as a PhD student soon after. Dame Wilson-Barnett later became professor of nursing at King's College London.

The inpatient wards at Guy's were based at the York Clinic, which was the first inpatient psychiatric unit

Reflections on the Challenges of Psychiatry in the UK and Beyond
© Pavilion Publishing and Media Ltd and its licensors 2017.

attached to a teaching hospital in the UK. Professor Edgar Jones, who completed a PhD at Guy's, wrote about its history:

'...the York Clinic at Guy's Hospital set up in April 1944 by Air Commodore Robert Gillespie. Gillespie had trained at the Cassel Hospital and Johns Hopkins, Baltimore, before being appointed physician in psychological medicine at Guy's in 1926. Recruited into the air force on the outbreak of war, he was posted to the RAF Officers' Hospital, Torquay, to investigate the nature of breakdown among aircrew. The experience of treating men with no history of mental illness and who did not fall into the traditional asylum diagnoses led Gillespie to consider social and cultural factors in the causation and treatment of psychoneuroses... were from the armed forces, the majority being diagnosed as anxiety states and 'combat exhaustion coming a good second'. Treatment was broadly-based including continuous baths, narcosis and ECT for the most disturbed patients and occupational (leather work, carpentry and model making) and individual therapy for milder cases... Social activity was identified as 'one of the most important therapeutic agents': 'the patients ... elect committees to organize weekly dances, charades, musical evenings, debates, and games tournaments'. Although not specifically a therapeutic community, the liberal regime and range of treatments offered marked a change from the asylum culture and represented a conscious attempt to raise the status of psychiatry and its allied disciplines. Following the suicide of Gillespie in October 1945, Thomas A Munro, recently returned from military service in India,

became the York Clinic's second director. It became part of the NHS in 1948 when fifteen of the forty-one beds were allocated to the health service. The atmosphere of the clinic was described by J J Fleminger, who arrived in 1955 to find: "… a compact unit on a 'domestic scale' where a relatively small staff knew each other well … The sister in charge of the York Clinic entertained us to tea with sandwiches and cakes every afternoon at half-past three. The York Clinic had its own kitchen and chef … It was all not merely comfortable—it was charming."[6]

The York Clinic was still very friendly and charming at the time I first arrived there in 1975. Coffee was still served in the staff common room in the morning and after lunch, and tea in the afternoon with occasional cakes! The York Clinic had its own parking that was used by staff members, with the daily presence of the green Volkswagen van of Jim Watson, and later the Rolls-Royce of Professor Elaine Murphy, taking up a lot of parking space. There was a tendency for all of us working at the York Clinic to have lunch together, sitting at one large table in the main staff restaurant in the nursing home. Many informal discussions took place in these gatherings, which were very helpful. This contributed to the significant degree of cohesion among members of staff and was missed as community care developed, when the hospital stopped being everyone's point of reference and staff members were dispersed all over the locality.

Soon after Jim Watson arrived as professor at Guy's, one of the inpatient wards at the York Clinic became a modified therapeutic community and adopted

6   Jones E (2004) War and the practice of psychotherapy: The UK experience 1939–1960. *Medical History* **48** (4) 493–510.

a 'social therapy approach'. It was run by Jim and Bernie Rosen. Authority was delegated from medical staff to colleagues in other disciplines to a substantial degree and also to patients themselves, although senior doctors retained ultimate responsibility for inpatients. Some patients were almost entirely treated by non-medical professionals. As far as possible, treatment plans were negotiated in contract meetings involving the patient and members of staff, who might be doctors, psychologists, nurses or social workers. Every patient was expected to participate fully in daily group activities, unless their treatment programme explicitly excluded this. A large community meeting took place once a week and most of the staff involved with patients' treatment attended. Patients received medication as appropriate, but emphasis was placed on psychological treatment methods. The orientation was eclectic, with emphasis on time-limited 'here and now' therapies, including behavioural and marital psychotherapies. Admissions, but not necessarily discharges, were medical decisions. The junior doctor and nurses did not wear uniform.

Another ward was run on traditional medical model lines run by the consultant psychiatrist Dr John Fleminger. Authority resided with medical staff, with an explicit hierarchy of responsibility from the top downwards. The most junior doctor wore a white coat and had medical responsibility for patients whose psychiatric problems were dealt with by the senior psychiatrist. Nurses wore uniforms and took a traditional nursing approach towards the patients.

Patients were treated in bed on admission, physical methods of treatment were often used, and 'good doctoring' was highly valued. Patients' progress was assessed in ward rounds where multidisciplinary consultation contributed to the formulation of the treatment. Group meetings were not held and most patients who were not on bed rest engaged in prescribed occupational therapy activities. Admission, discharge and treatment were medical decisions.

The comparison of these two contrasting inpatient psychiatric wards became the subject of my PhD thesis. I examined patients' disturbed behaviour and dissatisfaction with the ward atmosphere, and the correlation between those two factors and patient's personal and social variables such as gender, diagnosis, personality traits and length of stay in hospital. The methodology for the study included the use of instruments, some of them self-devised, to measure daily and weekly disturbed behaviour, weekly dissatisfaction and staff changes including members of staff leaving or going on holidays. This study was the first of a series taking place in the academic Department of Psychiatry at Guy's and attracted the interest of other colleagues. Sometimes some persuasion was needed to enable them to provide the necessary information, as most of them were not used to participating in research studies. Billy Goviden, charge nurse at the time, was most helpful in persuading his colleagues to participate willingly in the research.

In the meantime, my clinical experience at Guy's was thought-provoking and exciting. I attended several of the activities in different wards; outpatient clinics; and the rapidly increasing academic programme of lectures, workshops, and special interests activities such as psychotherapy, family therapy, marital therapy and psychosexual problems clinic. This last was among the first in the country, initiated by Jim Watson and the clinical psychologist Maurice Yaffe, who unfortunately was lost very young.

Huge amounts of data were collected for my study over a period of 75 weeks and 170 patients and this required computerised analysis. There was at Guy's the 'computer unit' with very bulky equipment that operated using the old type of punch cards, a system that was extremely time consuming. The staff at the unit were very helpful but also very busy with other projects. Except for Tom Trauer, we all had a limited knowledge of statistics. I was very fortunate that Clair Chilvers, senior lecturer in statistics at the School of Hygiene and Tropical Medicine in London, was brought in by Professor Stewart Cameron to help with the medical statistics of the embryonic research of the time at Guy's. Clair Chilvers later held several distinguished academic positions, including professor of epidemiology at the University of Nottingham, director of the mental health research and development portfolio at the Department of Health, director of the National Forensic Mental Health R&D Programme, and founder trustee of Mental Health Research UK. Her assistance in the analysis of data was crucial. She sent all of us to a Statistical Package for the Social Sciences (SPSS) course run by the University of London. Until then none of us, including the operators of the computer unit at Guy's, were using the SPSS. She also directed us to a free punching card service, again at the University of London, which was of great help. It was a relief not to be punching all the data alone, and it saved me a lot of time! The analysis of data lasted several months and the assistance of Tom Trauer and Clair Chilvers, was invaluable. The results showed that different types of ward environment affected patients' behaviour in different ways. Patients were more disturbed in the therapeutic community ward than in the conventional medical ward. Using a mathematical model, a relationship was demonstrated between ward model, type of behavioural disturbance and psychiatric diagnosis. Patients with the diagnosis schizophrenia tended to be more disturbed than other patients. In addition, by using a time-series analysis, the level of disturbed behaviour during a week was shown to be related to the level of disturbance during the preceding and following weeks; thus the levels of ward disturbance could be predicted.

I successfully defended my PhD Thesis, entitled *The Disturbed Behaviour of Patients in Psychiatric Wards*, in 1979. I still remember how the external examiner Professor Robin Priest of St Mary's Hospital Medical School in London announced the outcome of the examiners' deliberation. He said: 'Dr Bouras we have four choices: first, to fail you, second, to ask you to resubmit your thesis with major revisions, third, to ask you to resubmit the thesis with minor revisions and fourth, to pass you as it stands – and we have decided on the last one.' I felt that was a cruel way to let me know that I had passed my viva!

Once I had completed the two years registration for my PhD and while I carried out the statistical analysis and writing-up of my thesis I was offered a registrar post, to gain some clinical experience, at the psychiatric unit of St Olave's District General Hospital in Bermondsey, which was affiliated with Guy's. Dr Raghu Gaind and Dr Anthony Fry were the consultant psychiatrists there. I worked for six months with Dr Gaind and acquired valuable experience of acute inpatient psychiatry. At the same time, I worked at the Day Hospital, which was an entirely new entity for me. We published, with the head nursing colleague Richard Kember, an article in *Nursing Times* describing the utilisation of the facility, the pattern of organisation and function, and the demographic and clinical characteristics of the patients who attended the day hospital over the period of a year.

When the six months were up I rotated to Guy's as a registrar for the emergency psychiatric department, known then as 'casualty'. I had a very quiet first day with my new duties, working at the computer unit and analysing data for my thesis, until I was about to hand over the emergency bleep to the evening on-call psychiatrist. Then suddenly my bleep started ringing constantly. Once I found a telephone to answer the bleep, which was necessary in that time before mobile phones, I realised that something serious had happened. The switchboard operator, almost shouting, instructed me to rush to the maternity ward. When I arrived there I found pandemonium, with several policemen, some of them sitting on a man on the floor, surrounded by broken glass and there was panic among staff and patients. The ward sister explained to me that the man whom the police were holding on the floor had been told that his wife had given birth to a baby with Down's syndrome. He had reacted by throwing chairs against the windows smashing the glass. He had since then calmed down and I spoke to him. He was very distressed when he was told the condition of his newly born baby and 'did not know what he was doing'. I was not able to elicit symptoms of a psychiatric illness, except acute stress, hence the dilemma of what to do with him? The ward staff put pressure on me to admit him to the psychiatric unit at Guy's because they were afraid that if he was let free he might come back to the ward putting staff and patients at risk. The psychiatric unit at Guy's would not accept him because of the degree of his violent behaviour and the fact that he did not have a psychiatric illness. The efforts to find a satisfactory solution took several hours and eventually I arranged with the on-call psychiatrist at Bexley Psychiatric Hospital to accept him on a Section 136 of the then Mental Health Act. Section 136 required 'the police to transfer a person to a place of safety for psychiatric assessment'. This was a desperate decision but I felt that I had no other options available. The next day he was discharged by the consultant psychiatrist at Bexley Hospital. That was my turbulent first experience of the psychiatric casualty department at Guy's.

The psychiatric registrar post at the emergency department at Guy's also included dealing with first-line liaison referrals from the medical and surgical wards. I stayed at that position for six months and introduced some operational changes. It became obvious to me that many psychiatric emergencies were related to social factors, and I suggested that it would be helpful to have access to a social worker to carry out joint assessments with me. Tony Siegal, a psychiatric social worker, was assigned to the emergency psychiatric department and we worked closely together. We initiated a regular weekly clinical meeting involving us from psychiatry but also medical, nursing and admin staff from the emergency department. We reviewed the records of patients seen during working hours from Monday to Friday over a period of six months, and found that there was a dramatic increase in referrals by GPs compared to previous years and the admission rate was as high as 34% – I had been influenced by conducting my PhD research, and in whatever position I was placed, I tried to look at factual data. I enjoyed this post and found the experience very helpful and at the end of the six-month assignment I was requested to stay on for another six months. The reason for this was that the psychiatric unit at St Olave's Hospital had to close and all inpatient psychiatric services were going to be transferred to Guy's to occupy the inpatient medical and surgical wards space vacated from the closure of part of the hospital. These were effects of the reorganisation of the NHS taking place in the late 1970s and early 1980s. Physicians and surgeons at Guy's were very unhappy with the closure of their wards but even more unhappy with the psychiatric services moving in!

In the meantime, under the leadership of Jim Watson the academic Department of Psychiatry at Guy's was expanding dramatically. The undergraduate teaching was organised by Bernie Rosen, senior lecturer in psychiatry, and more and more senior colleagues were joining, mostly in an honorary capacity, as part of their clinical work with the NHS. Research was also growing in different directions. I was asked to support colleagues doing research because I was among the few psychiatrists at Guy's at the time who had research knowledge and experience. In that capacity I was involved in clinical trials of using trazodone and bromocriptine in depression, with Dr Paul Bridges who had a special interest in refractory depression. Paul Bridges also carried out assessments on patients with severe chronic depression for psychosurgery at the Neurosurgery Unit at the Brook Hospital in Shooters Hill, South East London. In 1980 Dr Maurice Lipsedge, a psychiatrist well known for his transcultural psychiatry interest and co-author with Roland Littlewood of the book *Aliens and Alienists* joined the academic and clinical psychiatric department at Guy's and I was assigned as his first registrar.

With the completion of my PhD it was time to organise my return to Greece and my colleagues in Athens were making various suggestions to me for jobs. I met with Jim Watson and told him my intention to leave for Greece. His answer was to stay a little longer in Britain and to consider a research position at a new Community Mental Health Centre in Lewisham called the Mental Health Advice Centre (MHAC). This was discussed with Dr Douglas Brough, consultant psychiatrist, who was the director of the MHAC. Douglas phoned me at home the same evening and invited me to start as senior research registrar at the MHAC as soon as possible. This offer posed a

great personal and family dilemma: should we leave
for Greece or stay longer and have the advantage of
experience in the new emerging trends of community
psychiatry? My wife Maria had completed her MSc
degree in town planning at the London School of
Economics and had started a part-time job at the
Development and Planning Unit at University College
London. Our twin daughters Christine and Irene were
about to start school and we had already registered
them with the English school in Athens. At the same
time, we were feeling integrated in London, having
made several friends professionally and socially.

I felt that the 1970s and 1980s were an electrifying
period of British psychiatry. Dynamic new ideas,
promising new service developments, optimism from
new treatment methods, research and the prospect of
community care were some of the promising aspects
of British psychiatry at that time. At Guy's, Jim
Watson was taking any opportunity to expand the
department academically and clinically, by adding
different psychiatric specialties as well as psychologists,
nurses, therapists and social workers all working in
a multidisciplinary context still based in the hospital
setting. There was a very supportive and friendly
climate at work with very exciting innovations taking
place, such as the introduction of nurse therapists,
the growing psychosexual problems clinic, cognitive
analytical therapy (CAT) introduced by Anthony
Ryle, etc.[7] Trainees were completing the training

---

7   Esteemed psychiatric colleagues such as Raghu Gaind, Antony
    Fry, Paul Bridges, Maurice Lipsedge, and later Elaine Murphy, the
    first woman professor of psychiatry of old age in England; Tom
    Craig, the first professor of community psychiatry in England; and
    Tony Cox, professor of child and adolescent psychiatry joined the
    academic department at Guy's, together with clinical psychologists
    Tom Trauer, John Weinman, Maurice Yaffe, Stan Newman, Evelyn
    Hendry and several others, most of whom became lifelong friends.

scheme and being appointed as consultants in various places around the South East region or elsewhere, strengthening the links of their local departments with Guy's. Furthermore, there was the promising prospect of community care with the exciting development of the MHAC in Lewisham.

In addition to these developments, I had started writing up and publishing articles, mostly from my PhD and other clinical studies that I was involved with. The following incident from the publication of one of the first articles is worth mentioning as it reflects some of the attitudes of the time. In an article that I co-authored with Clair Chilvers, Jim Watson and Tom Trauer, we described the mathematical model to predict the patients' disturbed behaviour in the wards that I had studied in my PhD. We submitted it for publication to *Psychological Medicine*, a journal of high reputation even before the introduction of the impact factor, and we received the comments of the reviewers for revisions. There were, however, some additional comments by the editor Michael Shepherd, professor of psychiatric epidemiology at the Institute of Psychiatry, that none of us were able to understand. Jim Watson, who knew Michael Sheppard from his time at the Maudsley, made an appointment for us to see Michael and ask his clarification. While we were leaving Guy's for the Maudsley, having waited for several weeks for this appointment, we received a call from Michael Sheppard cancelling our meeting. At the insistence of Jim Watson that we only wanted to ask him one question for two minutes he agreed to see us and as soon as we entered his office he greeted us by saying, 'I understand it's only one question for two minutes!' That was it. The paper was published and we were inundated with requests for reprints (as this was how papers were disseminated before the internet). There was still a lot of interest in improving the ward environment of psychiatric wards before the era of community care.[8]

We resolved our family dilemma by deciding to extend our stay in London and gain more professional experience. As it transpired, that extended stay would last over 40 years; we are still here to this day.

---

8   Bouras N, Chilvers C & Watson J P (1984) Estimating levels of disturbed behaviour among psychiatric inpatients using a general linear model. *Psychological Medicine* **14** (2) 439–444.

Chapter 2: Mental Health Advice Centre

On 1 April 1981 I arrived at the Mental Health Advice Centre (MHAC) as senior research registrar. I was tasked with consolidating and expanding the research activity that had already been started a year earlier by the psychiatrist Dr Rosalind Furlong, senior registrar at the time, who was moving on in her career. The centre became an 'off shore' research unit of the Guy's Department of Psychiatry. In addition to my involvement in the evaluation of the MHAC, the psychiatrist Dr Sourangshu Acharyya had started a project exploring the role of the psychiatrist in the multidisciplinary team, and the clinical psychologist Sandra Elliot was looking at postnatal emotions.

The MHAC was started informally in 1976 by Douglas Brough, consultant psychiatrist for the Borough of Lewisham in South East London, together with a small team of mental health professionals who developed a limited domiciliary based project for psychiatric assessment and treatment. Douglas Brough at that time had a long-standing involvement with the Department of Health, known then as the Department of Health and Social Security (DHSS). The only psychiatric services available locally before the MHAC were twice-weekly services for outpatients, and these were housed in a portakabin in Lewisham

Hospital. The admission inpatient beds were in Bexley Hospital, a psychiatric hospital miles away. Douglas Brough was a charismatic psychiatrist who foresaw that mental health services were moving rapidly towards community care. Thus he took the initiative to set up the MHAC in his catchment area in Lewisham in South East London. He received a generous grant from the Gatsby Charitable Foundation of the Sainsbury Family Trusts, whose chairman was David Sainsbury.[9]

The MHAC started operating formally in November 1978 from a large Victorian house in Handen Road and provided a new way of delivering mental health services in the late 1970s. The building had a bright yellow door and the centre became known as the 'Yellow Door' as well as 'Open Door'. It served a diverse catchment area with a population of 84,000. The aim was to integrate primary healthcare with mental health services and to provide easy access for patients to psychiatric and psychological help in the community, by making the MHAC the main portal of entry to the secondary care system. There was added value as the MHAC was linked with the academic Department of Psychiatry at Guy's and an evaluation process was built in by Jim Watson from the beginning. The staff of the MHAC consisted of a multidisciplinary team of psychiatrists, clinical psychologists, community psychiatric nurses, an occupational therapist, social workers, a psychotherapist and an administrator. One of the innovations was that patients could simply 'walk in' without having been referred by their GP or another community agent. There was a group of volunteers supporting the MHAC and a League of Friends chaired by the renowned actress Glenda Jackson, a local resident then living

---

9   David Sainsbury became Minister of Sciences and Innovation from 1998 to 2006 with the Labour Government of Tony Blair. He is currently Baron Sainsbury of Turville.

in Greenwich. It was soon realised that a number of emergency cases (usually patients with psychosis) were not able to reach the MHAC and a second team, the Crisis Intervention Team (CIT), was formed. This team was also multidisciplinary and responded rapidly to calls by general practitioners by going out to see people in their homes, at police stations, in hospital emergency departments, etc. The aims of the CIT were to provide quick and effective intervention for crisis situations and psychiatric emergencies, facilitate resolution of the acute situation and, if possible, avoid hospitalisation by providing treatment and support at home. The CIT was supported by psychiatric trainees from Guy's; Dr Mike Hobbs was the first and was succeeded by Dr Gwen Tufnell and later Dr Liz Parker. Later, a mental health rehabilitation function was added at the MHAC for people with long-standing mental health problems. In essence, the MHAC, with its walk-in crisis intervention and rehabilitation functions, was the predecessor of modern mental health services in the UK as we now know them – their implementation having started almost 20 years after the MHAC was established.

During the early days of the MHAC, a very large amount of data had been collected, which needed analysis and presentation. With the support of a research clerical assistant, the research procedure was reorganised and the data analysis was started. We had to punch thousands of cards and to use the computer unit at Guy's, which I had mastered using the SPSS. The first report, describing the MHAC's first three years of operation, was published in May 1982. It was a descriptive account of the work of the MHAC and was widely distributed nationally and internationally. The main findings showed an increase of self-referrals ('walk-ins') over the study period (the main diagnosis was adjustment disorder on the ICD-9 classification system in use at the time), while there was no reduction in inpatient psychiatric admissions. This report attracted remarkable interest from psychiatric colleagues, other mental health professionals and policy makers. It was the first comprehensive publication describing the development, structure and delivery of a community mental health service in the UK. We received a plethora of letters, mostly of support, and we were visited by many colleagues from different parts of the country and abroad who wanted to look at the MHAC and learn more about its structure and operation, its funding sources, and the prospects of further developments. Most of the professors of psychiatry in England at that time visited the MHAC, as well as many senior clinicians, for whom we organised special presentations.

Soon after the publication of the first report we published a second report referring to the work of the CIT, which showed that there were differences with the patients seen at the walk-in clinic. Most of those seen by the CIT had a diagnosis of schizophrenia and had a previous psychiatric history with inpatient admission and recent discontinuation of taking their medication. Those seen at the walk-in clinic had the diagnoses of adjustment disorder, anxiety and depression.

We were pleased with the response to our first report and shortly after, in 1982, we published a brief article in *Health Trends*, an official publication of the DHSS on public health issues. We were also invited to publish an article in the *Psychiatric Bulletin* of the Royal College of Psychiatrists and to make a presentation in the Maudsley Bequest lecture series at the Royal College of Psychiatrists' annual conference. The presentation was made jointly by Douglas Brough and Jim Watson at a session chaired by Anthony Clare, the Maudsley psychiatrist who became famous from his radio and television programmes *In the Psychiatrist's Chair*. There were mixed responses to the presentation. Though the majority of the audience were complementary and in favour of the development of the MHAC, some, including Anthony Clare, expressed reservations, pointing out that such a model of mental health service seemed to look after the 'worried well' and perhaps diverted resources from people with severe mental illness. Professor Steven Hirsch, of Charing Cross Medical School, was critical of the methodology of our analysis and stated that we wrongly used the term 'evaluation', which he said should mean that one variable is compared against another one, which was not the case with the MHAC. We became careful with the terminology we used in future and adopted the term 'descriptive evaluation'. Several articles were published in peer-reviewed journals, including the *Journal of General Practice*, while we continued receiving invitations for presentations at conferences or academic meetings nationally and internationally. While I was involved with the research at the MHAC, I maintained my clinical commitments by running a weekly outpatient clinic at Lewisham Hospital and taking the weekly ward round of an acute admissions psychiatric ward at Bexley Hospital.

The principles of delivery of mental health services introduced by the MHAC were rapidly gaining acceptance and community mental health care became the preferred model of care that over the years was gradually adopted all over the world with different variations. Following our work at the MHAC, the Gatsby Charitable Foundation decided to fund a national unit focused on community mental health research. There were discussions and deliberations as to how and where such a unit should be placed, and eventually it was awarded to Douglas Brough and Jim Watson. In 1985 the new unit, named the National Unit for Psychiatric Research and Development (NUPRD), was inaugurated with Dr Tom Craig, consultant psychiatrist, as the first director. The NUPRD was first housed in offices in the old nursing wing of the Lewisham Hospital. In 1989 it was renamed Research and Development for Psychiatry (RDP) and moved into offices at Borough High Street near London Bridge. RDP eventually became the Sainsbury Centre for Mental Health in February 1992, with Dr Matt Muijen, psychiatrist, as director. Tom Craig moved on to the chair of community psychiatry at Guy's and St Thomas' and remained a core member of the academic Department of Psychiatry at Guy's until its merger with the Institute of Psychiatry (IoP), when he moved to the Health Service and Population Research (HSPR) Department there (see also Chapter 11). The Sainsbury Centre for Mental Health maintained its links with the Guy's academic Department of Psychiatry for a while, before moving to a different department of King's College London (KCL) and eventually becoming an independent entity. In 2013 the Gatsby Charitable Foundation withdrew funding and today the centre operates independently as the Centre for Mental Health.

In the meantime, the academic department of psychiatry at Guy's, as part of the United Medical and Dental Schools (UMDS) that included St Thomas' Hospital Medical School, continued growing swiftly with new appointments of clinical academics, linked with new specialist services such as old age psychiatry, child and adolescent psychiatry, psychotherapy and intellectual disabilities. There were always strong links with local mental health services in Southwark and Lewisham and later Lambeth, as well as with the extended South East Thames region for services and the organisation and running of the psychiatric training scheme. Research also grew remarkably in several areas, including psychopharmacology, liaison psychiatry, mental health problems in patients with cancer, psychotherapy with the development of cognitive analytic therapy (CAT), family and marital therapy and psychosexual problems. Prominence continued to be given to community mental health, particularly with the links with the MHAC and the NUPRD.

At the peak of the MHAC development in the summer of 1982, Dr Raghu Gaind, chairman of the Division of Psychiatry at that time, informed me that Guy's would soon be advertising a new consultant post as half-time in mental handicap – as it was then known, subsequently becoming learning disabilities (LD) and today intellectual disabilities (ID) – and half-time senior lecturer within the academic Department of Psychiatry at Guy's. Dr Gaind strongly advised me to apply for this post because of my strong community psychiatry background and also because services for people with ID were planned to become entirely community-based.

The opportunity to apply for a consultant post created new and more difficult personal and family dilemmas. First, I had no experience in mental handicap. In fact, when I was involved with the emergency psychiatric service at Guy's I had many difficulties in dealing with people with mental handicap as there were no local services and the system of care was very confusing. Second, we were actively looking to return to Greece, as we were under pressure from our families and from colleagues who were suggesting appealing jobs to us. The prospect of gaining more experience in London as a consultant psychiatrist was very tempting. The decision was that I would apply for the post and if I was successful my family and I would extend our stay in London for a while. This was the advice of all senior colleagues with the exception of Douglas Brough, who was not happy at my leaving the MHAC. I had been presenting a paper about the MHAC at the Ninth International Congress of Social Psychiatry in Paris, and had to return to London in a hurry for the consultant's interview the next day. I was offered the consultant post in mental handicap, half-time, on the grounds that although I had no experience in that field, the service was going to be radically reorganised based on community care where I had already developed expertise. The other half-time of my appointment was as senior lecturer with the academic Department of Psychiatry at UMDS, which would allow me to continue to be involved with the research of the MHAC.

I was succeeded at the MHAC by the psychiatrist Dr Jed Boardman, with whom I had worked for several years, documenting the work of the MHAC in articles published in peer-reviewed journals and research reports. The contribution of Jed strengthened the evidence base of the MHAC and opened new directions for the development of community psychiatry. I had known Jed since he was a medical student at Guy's when he had led the Issues in Healthcare Group, which organised talks and debates. Among the speakers were Keith Joseph, Lord David Owen and Vincente Navarro, professor of public health at Johns Hopkins University in Baltimore, one of the most charismatic speakers I have ever heard. Jed Boardman latterly became well known for his work on primary care, psychosocial aspects of mental health and the employment of service users. In the meantime, the MHAC, in addition to the walk-in clinic and the CIT, developed a rehabilitation team in 1983 to deal with the rehabilitation problems of individuals with chronic schizophrenia in the catchment area. All in all, the MHAC provided a compelling early example of policy implications in the rapidly growing

Reflections on the Challenges of Psychiatry in the UK and Beyond
© Pavilion Publishing and Media Ltd and its licensors 2017.

field of community mental health care and the complex operational issues involved with the implementation of different community care programmes. Douglas Brough retired in 1984 and the MHAC moved to new premises in Southbrook Road in Lee, South East London, in 1986, where it has continued to operate until the present day as a catchment area community mental health team (CMHT). The MHAC was certainly ahead of its time.

Chapter 3:
Consultant psychiatrist

I took up my consultant post in October 1982 on
the expectation that I would apply the emerging
new ideas of community psychiatry to a strongly
institutionalised and stagnated service system that
needed urgent reforms. This system was made up of
the institutions for people with intellectual disabilities
(ID). Because of my lack of experience in ID, my
appointment was proleptic for six months, with the
obligation to attend the clinical and academic activities
of Professor Joan Bicknell's department. Joan Bicknell
was the first professor of mental handicap and was
based at St George's Hospital Medical School, South
West London, where the chairman of the academic
department of psychiatry was Professor Arthur Crisp,
a renowned world expert in eating disorders. Joan
Bicknell was a charismatic clinician and teacher and
was devoted to improving the quality of services for
people with ID. Her book *The Psychopathology of
Mental Handicap* is a classic. I attended her clinical
work at St Ebba's Hospital, a long-stay institution for
people with ID in Surrey, and the academic meetings
at St George's Hospital Medical School. It was a
very interesting and helpful introduction to a field
of psychiatry that I did not know. Sophie Thomson,
senior registrar in psychiatry at that time, was among
the core members of the clinical team. I began to

understand the policy context and the political aspects involved in that area of ID. I maintained regular links with Joan Bicknell until her retirement, and continued to do so with her successor, Sheila Hollins, as well as with other colleagues in the St George's department.[10]

There had been two major public enquires about the appalling conditions in the asylums for people with ID at Ely Hospital in 1969 and Normansfield Hospital in 1979. In response to growing concern and the outcomes of the public enquiry into Ely Hospital, in 1971 the government had published the white paper *Better Services for the Mentally Handicapped*, which made recommendations for the closure of the long-stay institutions and the development of community care services. A few years before, President John F. Kennedy's administration in the USA had enabled key legislation such as the Maternal and Child Health and Mental Retardation Planning Amendments (1963) and The Mental Retardation Facilities and Community Mental Health Centres Construction Act (1963). These policies paved the way in the USA for the beginning of the early deinstitutionalisation programmes. University Affiliate Programs (professional training, research and service centres) were established, as well as Mental Retardation Research Centres, and the National Institute of Child Health and Human Development at the National Institutes. The Kennedy family had an interest in ID because Rosemary, one of the President's sisters, was born with mild ID and underwent a prefrontal lobotomy at the age 23, which left her permanently incapacitated. She was institutionalised at the Fort Atkinson Memorial Hospital in Wisconsin,

10 Sheila Hollins was professor of learning disability at St George's Hospital Medical School, president of the royal college of psychiatrists, 2005–2008; president of the British Medical Association, 2012–2013; and from 2010, Baroness Hollins of Wimbledon.

where she died at the age of 83 in 2005.

The New Frontier Program and the political consensus at that time in the US emphasised the universality of human rights that explicitly extended to disabled people in the later Declaration on the Rights of Disabled Persons and the later UN Declaration on the Rights of Disabled Persons and the Declaration on the Rights of Mentally Retarded Persons in 1971. Within democratic societies, politics became increasingly dominated by the demands for full social inclusion for racial and ethnic minorities, women and people with disabilities. Campaigns against the large institutions were supported by a series of enquiries into severe neglect and brutality taking place within them, and by research showing the disabling effect of life in a total institution, particularly Goffman's influential work in the 1960s.[11] Some of the first clinical effectiveness research in this field found that community-based units had better outcomes in terms of behaviour and self-care skills. Renewed therapeutic optimism led to services for people with ID increasingly recruiting clinical psychologists, educationalists, occupational therapists, and speech and language therapists, who for the most part had less personal investment in maintaining total institutions.

The move from institutional care was also promoted by a zealous movement based on 'normalisation theory'. This originated from Scandinavia and emphasised the need for each disabled person to develop a sense of self-worth and adulthood by experiencing and passing over the various thresholds of challenge and growth common to all people. The key role for public services was therefore to facilitate opportunities for disabled people

---

11 Bouras N (2014) On asylums: Essays on the social situation of mental patients and other inmates by Erving Goffman. *British Journal of Psychiatry* **205** 407.

to experience the same kinds of living environment as the general population, with similar opportunities for self-determination, personal and sexual relationships, and earning a living. Facilitation essentially involved compensating for a person's disabilities, such as providing staff to support a disabled person in carrying out domestic tasks or specialised transport to help them get to town. Normalisation theory was promoted in services for people with ID by the influential writings of Wolf Wolfensberger and his evaluation system PASS (Programme Analysis of Service Systems). Wolfensberger pointed out the need to overcome the social psychology of discrimination.[12] He noted that disabled people suffer disadvantages not only in the form of overt discrimination, but also by an unconscious process of denigration, and he observed how specialist services used derogatory labels or associated disabled people with other groups with a low status in society. This confirmed to disabled people their inferior and dependent position in society, which they in turn expressed through their behaviour, thereby confirming the initial assumptions of their lower status. He proposed that a key objective of services should therefore be to enable disabled people to behave in ways that are socially valued rather than inferior, in order to assert their equal status and achieve acceptance by others in society. This, he proposed, could be attained by making staff aware of the ways in which they and their workplaces could unconsciously devalue disabled people, by making every effort to place disabled people in positive social roles and to help them behave and appear in ways that are socially valued, by helping them develop their personal competencies, and by ensuring they take part in social activities in their community. This involves living in 'normative housing within the valued community with

---

12 Wolfensberger W (1991) Reflections on a lifetime in human services and mental retardation. *Mental Retardation* **29** (1) 1–16.

valued people', attending the same schools, and being involved in a valued manner in work, shopping and leisure activities.

Wolfensberger later introduced a similar concept, namely 'social role valorisation'. Wolfersberger's writings about normalisation theory, social role valorisation and 'citizen advocacy' accompanied by the evaluation methodologies embraced in *Program Analysis of Service Systems* (PASS) and *Program Analysis of Service Systems Implementation of Normalisation Theory Goals* (PASSING), offered a way to identify and discuss fundamental aspects of a quality service. There was, however, little sound theory or scientific evidence to support this vision, either in terms of rational development or institutional change. With some exceptions, psychiatrists remained reserved and sceptical.[13] Reservations notwithstanding, the normalisation theory principle captured the imagination and commitment of many professionals, service planners, service providers and others. Normalisation theory workshops were led by charismatic individuals whose vision about how to revolutionise human services became contagious. Some psychologists were numbered among the leading advocates. There is no doubt that over the next few decades every policy initiative for people with mental handicap, or intellectual and developmental disabilities explicitly stated its commitment to the principle of normalisation theory. Normalisation theory – along with the 'five accomplishments' of John O' Brien: community presence, relationships, choice, competence and respect – dominated all aspects of planning services for people with ID. In the implementation of plans the dominant concept was planning for individual needs (PIN). The

13 Bouras N & Ikkos G (2013) Ideology, psychiatric practice and professionalism. *Psychiatriki* **24** (1) 17–27.

dominance of normalisation theory in clinical practice and service developments was not without problems. An interesting critique of the principles of normalisation theory, as perceived by a young psychiatrist during her training with us, was published by Dr Anne Boucherat.[14]

Normalisation theory started being implemented in various model services, of which the most influential was that of the Eastern Nebraska Community Office of Retardation (ENCOR). This service pioneered the adaptation of ordinary houses to provide staff supported residences for small groups of people with ID, together with a small staff team. In the UK, this model inspired the report by the King's Fund, *An Ordinary Life*,[15] which came at the moment when changes in social security regulations provided a substantial expansion of public funds for resettling people from long-stay hospital care into the community.[16] *An Ordinary Life* stated that people with ID should live in ordinary houses in community streets, with the same range of choices as any citizens and mixing as equals with other members of the community.

In such a complex international policy environment, the views of the psychiatric profession were rather blurred and their role was becoming poorly defined. In the UK, though, psychiatrists were critical about the condition in the institutions, while at the same time they had reservations about the feasibility of the proposed community care plans. In the 1970s the Royal College of Psychiatrists debated whether ID presented a psychiatric

14 Boucherat A (1987) Normalisation in mental handicap–acceptance without questions? *Bulletin of the Royal College of Psychiatrists* **11** 423.

15 King's Fund (1981) *An Ordinary Life*. London: King's Fund.

16 Cumella S (2007) Mental health and intellectual disabilities: The development of services. In: N Bouras and G Holt (eds) *Psychiatric and Behavioural Disorders in Intellectual and Developmental Disabilities*. Cambridge: Cambridge University Press.

speciality or not. The view that prevailed was that the role of the psychiatrist should be focused on addressing the mental health problems of people with ID and a speciality of 'psychiatry of mental handicap' should be established at the college. Among the pioneers were Drs Jose Jancar, Yvonne Wiley, Ken Day, Andrew Reid, Professor Joan Bicknell and others. Even between them, however, there were mixed views, and they were not in agreement about the implementation of community care plans. Clinical psychologists, nurses, therapists, social workers and various activists were clearer about what needed to be done and more enthusiastic in their support of the proposed community care plans.

At the centre of this policy context, in October 1982 I joined, as a consultant psychiatrist, the Project Team at Guy's for developing community services for adults with ID. The services for children with ID were separate and the responsibly of the Developmental Paediatrics Department at Guy's. The other members of the Project Team were Ann Bosanquet, administrator; Dot Wotton, nurse manager; Catherine Dooley, clinical psychologist; and Pauline Formby, secretary. Catherine Dooley also had no clinical experience in ID, only in adult general psychiatry, and we had worked together at St Olave's Hospital. My contractual responsibility was to spend half of my time working with the Project Team for the North Southwark catchment area, and to spend the other half teaching and doing research with the Academic Department of Psychiatry at Guy's Hospital Medical School. We were first based at the Royal Eye Hospital at St George's Circle, in one open office space in Southwark not far from Guy's. The Royal Eye Hospital was used at that time as the administration and management offices of the District Health Authority and was deliberately chosen to accommodate our Project Team to signify the separation of our service from hospitals, though it was an old, disused hospital and in fact the only available accommodation!

In 1981 the then Guy's Health District Management Team commissioned a development group, which was funded by the Guy's Hospital Special Trustees, to produce a report concerning 'mentally handicapped people' for Lewisham and North Southwark (the South Southwark area was the responsibility of the Maudsley Hospital). The Development Group consisted of Alan Tyne, Ann Bosanquet and Bill Mitchell. Alan Tyne was well known nationally for his involvement in a charity pressure group at the time known as Campaign for Mental Handicap, which advocated for better services and the rights of people with ID. Bill Mitchell was a clinical psychologist.

The Development Group produced a detailed report that became known as the 'Orange Report' because it had an orange cover! The 'Orange Report' was based on the principles of normalisation theory with attention to the philosophy of the service that people with ID were equals in their human values and rights to all other people. The recommendations included client-centred services that should be coordinated, coherent, continuous and comprehensive. All the components of a community-based service for people with ID were described, including plans to resettle people from institutions in the community; development of community residential services for adults based on the 'core and cluster' model of the ENCOR scheme in Nebraska; day, evening and weekend respite services; family supports; multidisciplinary teams; special services; services for the most severely disabled people and those who had committed offences; proposals for research; and a rough estimate of the economic cost for all recommended services. The timescale for the full implementation of the plans was within 10 years. The 'Orange Report' attracted a lot of interest nationally and was highly sought for several years. It is not an exaggeration to note that the 'Orange Report', later becoming known as 'Orange Peril', represented an advanced vision of services for people with ID for that time and for the years to come.

Chapter 4: Developing the service

When the Project Group started working, the services for people with ID in the Guy's catchment area of North Southwark and North Lewisham were meagre. (The population in Lewisham was 238,000 and in North Southwark was 81,500.) There was Crispin House, an 'adult training centre' (ATC) run by Southwark Social Services and providing day care. Dr R. Rosenberg, consultant psychiatrist, undertook regular service users' reviews there in close collaboration with social services. He was employed by the South East Thames Region Health Authority (SETRHA) and assigned to the borough of Southwark, while the inpatient beds were at Darenth Park Hospital, a large institution in Kent with long-stay beds and short-stay admissions when they were required. In the borough of Lewisham there were two ATCs – Leemore and Mulberry – four residential facilities – Rokeby House, St Donatt's, Tresillian Road and Clarendon Rise – and the Grove Park Hospital in Lee with 168 long-stay beds, of which 99 were for the Bromley borough. The consultant psychiatrist for Lewisham, based at Grove Park Hospital, was Dr Peter Woolf, again employed by SETRHA, who had a traditional hospital-based mode of operation.

One of the first decisions made by the Project Group was not to try pilot schemes, but instead to develop new community-based services for people with ID for the whole catchment area of Lewisham and North Southwark. The Project Group was soon renamed the Adult Health Mental Handicap Team (AHMT), and its first priority was to plan for the resettlement of people from Darenth Park to the local communities. There were 69 people from Lewisham and North Southwark in Darenth Park, with a wide range of disabilities and lengths of stay, who had to be resettled.

We identified first a house for four people to open in Lewisham, and this took many months to become operational. Very soon the pressure was mounting on the AHMT to produce a deliverable plan for the resettlement of all the people under our responsibility, as SETRHA intensified the plans for the closure of Darenth Park. In the meantime, stronger and stronger ideological and political views on ID services were prevailing. The 'core and cluster' model for residential care was revised in favour of the concept of 'ordinary housing' that had been introduced by the King's Fund. Normalisation theory principles were fully adopted, sometimes to a rather extreme level. Nurses were out in favour of 'support workers'. On a personal level, I was under increasing pressure from adult psychiatry colleagues to take over the clinical care of people who had been historically or by default under their care. GPs and social services also started making referrals. I was a single-handed consultant within a planning team, and I was only able to respond at a consultative level with limited clinical responsibility; obviously, I was unable to take over inpatients without having any such facilities. I suggested starting an outpatient clinic but my proposal was rejected as 'representing the medical model'.

The Guy's Hospital setting

It is important to look at the management structures and professional surroundings of the AHMT at that time. We had good support from the then Guy's Hospital Health District, as it was known, and both Peter Griffiths, district administrator and Graham Winyard, district medical officer, were very supportive of the plans for developing community-based services for people with ID. Both later reached top positions in the NHS hierarchy, with Peter Griffiths becoming deputy chief executive for the Management Executive at the Department of Health and later heading the Health Quality Service. He was also the Chief Executive of the Guy's Hospital first-wave NHS Trust, which was termed a 'flagship' trust in the health service reforms of Margaret Thatcher's governments. Graham Winyard became deputy chief medical officer and medical director of the NHS in England, while playing a major role in the creation of the National Institute of Health and Care Excellence (NICE).

The same year of my appointment in 1982, the Guy's and St Thomas' Medical Schools merged to become United Medical and Dental Schools (UMDS). Also in 1982, Guy's Health District was merged with Lewisham Health District to form the Lewisham and North Southwark Health Authority. The implementation of the Roy Griffiths report in 1983 introduced the general management concept for responsible and accountable actions of an NHS body. This had profound effects on the running of the NHS, which inevitably affected the work of the AHMT; the main emphasis in the NHS at that time was on hospitals, and we were in the business of closing hospitals! There was a need to promote the interdependencies between hospitals, primary and social care.

Guy's Hospital was established as a National Health Service Trust in 1990 and three years later in 1993 merged with St Thomas' Hospital to form the Guy's and St Thomas' Hospital NHS Trust. This included the AHMT, which until then had been in a priority care unit together with mental health services and community services. Guy's Hospital included influential medical figures of high esteem, such as the Medical Director Sir Cyril Chantler; Paediatric Nephrologist Professor Maurice Lessof, an international authority on food allergy; and Professor Harry Keen, pioneer in the field of diabetes and staunch defender of the NHS who was instrumental in securing a judicial review of the NHS reforms. Dr George Houston, the dean of Guy's Medical School, was highly respected by his colleagues and had a unique style of chairing the ad hoc committees for new consultants' appointments. There were also medical politicians involved, such as Lord Ian McColl, professor of surgery and special advisor on healthcare to the Prime Minister Margaret Thatcher, and Sir Gerard Vaughan, consultant child psychiatrist, who became Minister of Health in one of Margaret Thatcher's governments.

Working in such an environment with so many highly regarded colleagues and rapid organisational changes nationally and locally was very inspiring but also demanding. The concept of community care for people with ID was alien to my clinician colleagues at Guy's Hospital. Whenever I raised with them issues related to our developments they gave me the same answer: 'We are not taking a medical lead in the developments of mental handicap.' In other words, 'Thank you but nothing to do with us!' This could be further translated to, 'Don't ask for any extra resources; enough has been diverted from the medical services.' It was only Jim Watson, as professor of psychiatry,

Reflections on the Challenges of Psychiatry in the UK and Beyond
© Pavilion Publishing and Media Ltd and its licensors 2017.

who was able to understand and appreciate our efforts, but even he lost track at times with the proposed innovations and ideas, while always being supportive of our plans over the years and offering me personal advice and support on many occasions.

On reflection, I don't think that we were clear ourselves about the magnitude of the tasks we had undertaken. I recall vividly, even now writing this book, the grave reservations of consultant psychiatrists already working with people with ID when I first introduced to them the plans for the closure of the hospitals and the community developments. Ann Moss, chief nursing officer of psychiatry at the York Clinic at Guy's, was very unhappy with the idea of employing support workers and not nurses, and she made strong representations to me. She said, 'If the nurses go then the doctors will follow.'

The first general manager/director of the AHMT was Nan Karl, an American with previous experience in disability services in the US and a strong advocate of normalisation theory. The plans for the new community care developments in our district were shaped over the next ten years including the closure of and resettlement from Darenth Park, development of community mental handicap teams, and closure of and resettlement from Grove Park.

Chapter 5: Resettlement programme

Darenth Park Hospital

Darenth Park Hospital was founded in 1878 in Dartford, Kent, as Darenth School for 500 children with ID. In 1911 it became the Darenth Industrial Trading Colony; it was almost entirely self-sufficient in food production and the manufacture of everyday items through the ample supply of free labour. In 1936, it became Darenth Park Hospital, and by 1970 the population had grown to 1,500 adults and children with ID. The physical conditions in this vast, grim Victorian building were increasingly unacceptable by modern standards. In 1973 the Regional Health Board agreed to close Darenth Park following the publication of the White Paper *Better Services for the Mentally Handicapped* in 1971, which laid the foundations of the new policy of providing small community-based units to replace the large institutions.[17] In 1978 the Darenth Park Steering Group was set up by SETRHA to coordinate the closure of the institution by March 1988. The closure plan

---

17 Department of Health and Social Security (1971) *Better Services for the Mentally Handicapped*. London: HMSO.

divided the institution into receiving districts, with ours being Lewisham and North Southwark. Detailed 'hospital reduction control plans' were produced and money, known as a 'dowry,' would follow each resettled person to their receiving district. In 1984 there were 677 residents in Darenth Park, 69 of whom belonged to our district of Lewisham and North Southwark.

The final phase of the closure project was led by the charismatic and formidable Audrey Emerton, regional chief nursing officer. Audrey Emerton was very committed to the project. She took a personal interest in monitoring the developments and was greatly assisted by Jim Mansell and his colleagues who had established the Institute of Social and Applied Psychology of the University of Kent that became the Tizard Centre (see also Chapter 6).

The resettlement of the 69 residents from our district involved a great deal of planning, including assessing and re-assessing individual needs, and liaising with their families whenever possible as well as respective social services departments. The resettlement was successfully completed within the required timeframe to community-based staff-supported houses. These housed four to six residents and met their needs as far as possible. Many visits and assessments were carried out on site at Darenth Park, which was becoming increasingly physically uninhabitable. We sought the views of relatives and carers and developed the community houses in collaboration with social services, housing associations and voluntary organisations. A few local residents expressed some reservations about having a house for people with ID in their neighbourhood. We reassured them by explaining that these houses and their residents would be fully supported by staff – and our reassurance was accepted. We maintained NHS responsibility initially in the first few houses, but we transferred it later either to social services or other relevant organisations such as housing associations. The resettled people became ordinary residents, not patients, in the community; they were entitled to benefits and to be registered with their own local GP.

As part of the multidisciplinary approach, we carried out mental health assessments, both before and after resettlement, as required, and we instigated therapeutic interventions as necessary. There were difficulties in the resettlement of some individuals with ID and serious behavioural problems, whether or not a diagnosable psychiatric disorder was present. This was experienced by all services involved in resettlement programmes. In view of mounting concern about the difficulties of resettled people with behavioural problems, SETRHA produced a report in 1984 referring to special services needed with the closure of Darenth Park.[18] The working group that produced this report was chaired by Dr John Corbett, consultant child psychiatrist and director of Hilda Lewis Unit at the Royal Bethlem Hospital, nationally and internationally known in the field of ID; he later became professor in learning disabilities in Birmingham University Medical School.

This report recommended that 'certain groups of people, particularly those with severe behavioural disorders would require specialised services, organised on a regional basis and that initially four units might be required, combined with individual District Units'. Furthermore, the report made the following recommendations:

18 Mental Handicap Special Services (1984) *Report of the Regional Mental Handicap Working Party (Special Services)*. London: South East Thames Regional Health Authority.

'... those services for severely mentally handicapped people who are severely disturbed should in the future be provided on a District basis.'

'Those services for mildly mentally handicapped people who are severely disturbed should be provided on a sub-Regional basis linked to a Special Advisory Team.'

'That a Specialist Team be established to provide on a visiting basis an advisory and teaching service to assist those caring for mentally handicapped people with sensory handicaps.'

'Those adequate facilities should be provided at District level for people who are mentally ill and mentally retarded.'

On reflection, the recommendations of this report were sound and prophetic of the problems that were faced when institutions were closed and community services developed, of which a particularly difficult problem was the lack of inpatient mental health units. The report recommended for South East London the development of inpatient assessment units: one at Grove Park Hospital and the other at the Maudsley Hospital. The development of an inpatient assessment unit in Grove Park Hospital within our locality was firmly rejected by our district. There was a belief that establishing comprehensive community services there will be no need for admissions will end and that if they were ever required then generic mental health services would be used. In retrospect, this proved to be a major mistake and miscalculation, because it deprived our district of inpatient mental health facilities that were, unsurprisingly, needed after having closed two institutions, Darenth Park and Grove Park, despite having developed extensive community services.

Two of the recommendations from this report materialised, with the formation of the Special Development Team and the establishment of the Mental Impairment Evaluation and Treatment Service Unit (MIETS) at the Maudsley Hospital in the grounds of the Royal Bethlem Hospital. The Special Development Team was established by SETRHA in 1986 and was led by the psychologist Eric Emerson, professor of disability and health research at the Centre for Disability Research, Lancaster University (see also Chapter 6).[19] It was an advisory service to enable local services to create residential housing services for people with severe ID and severe behavioural problems. SETRHA established the MIETS unit in 1987 with a strong multidisciplinary clinical team consisting of consultant psychiatrists Tony Holland[20] and Lachlan Campbell, both of the new generation of psychiatry colleagues firmly oriented towards community services; Glynis Murphy[21] and Isobel Claire, clinical psychologists; Kay Beaumont, social worker; Eddie Chaplin, ward manager; and others. The MIETS unit had 13 beds and provided a psychiatric assessment and treatment service for adults who had mild ID and serious behavioural problems and/or psychiatric disorders. The MIETS unit was

---

19 See a series of articles which described the function of the Special Development Team: Emerson E, Cummings R, Hughes H *et al* (1988) Challenging behaviour and community services: Evaluation and overview. *Mental Handicap* **17** 194–107.

20 Tony Holland, professor of learning disabilities, became nationally and internationally known for his research in ID.

21 Glynis Murphy became professor of clinical psychology and disability at the Tizard Centre, University of Kent; co-editor of the *Journal of Applied Research in Intellectual Disability,* and is a past president of the International Association for the Scientific Study of Intellectual Disability.

independently evaluated in 1992 by the London School of Economics Community and Health Research Group who produced evidence that the Districts in SETRHA were not able to resettle a group of residents from Darenth Park without additional specialist services and frequently had to use private facilities, a tendency that increased with time (see also Chapters 8 and 9).[22] This evaluation classified the views of those responsible for providing local services for people with severe behavioural problems into three categories:

1. 'Removers' do not want to develop locally the competence to serve people with behaviour problems and they seek instead to place people who cannot be served locally in out-of-area private residential placements, often at a considerable expense.

2. 'Containers' seek to provide local services but try only to contain people in low-cost and therefore poorly staffed settings.

3. 'Developers' seek to provide local services that really do address individual needs, and therefore give higher priority to funding services that, with more staff, training and management input, are more expensive than ordinary community services.

We faced many clinical challenges in our district in the process of resettling residents in community placements. The following cases stand out in my memory even today. A young man with severe ID and severe self-injurious behaviour, who was kept in the notorious Ward 19 of Darenth Park – 'the disturbed ward' – absorbed much team consideration in planning to meet his needs in a community house. He was eventually resettled in

22 Dockrell G, Gaskell G & Rehman H (1992) *Community Care and Challenging Behaviour: Practices and policies: The MIETS evaluation*. London: London School of Economics Community and Health Research Group.

a staff-supported house in Lewisham on his own, at the recommendation of the Special Development Team. This did not prove a successful arrangement in spite of high financial cost and the admirable efforts of his very committed support workers and various psychological and psychiatric interventions. Two other residents with mild ID, a psychiatric diagnosis of psychosis and a criminal history also presented serious challenges for their resettlement. Neither fitted into the services we developed and were more suitable for generic adult mental health services, which refused to accept them. Finally, after many efforts, we admitted them to the MIETS unit, where they had a very long admission and assessment period until eventually our district generic adult mental health services accepted responsibility and the service users were transferred to them. For using the Special Development Team and MIETS our budget was top-sliced, which meant losing local funding to a regional service outside our control, much to our displeasure. We felt strongly that there was no substitute for the development of local services with local accountability and self-sufficiency. Though both these regional services made valuable contributions in the development of comprehensive community services, no firm conclusions of their effectiveness were drawn and no controlled evaluation studies were carried out.

The closure of Darenth Park was finally completed in August 1988, when the last residents were transferred and the asylum finally shut its doors. Darenth Park was the first large regional mental handicap institution to close in the UK as a result of government policy. The process of the closure project was described in an interesting book entitled *Hospital Closure*.[23] We also documented our involvement from a clinical perspective,

23 Korman N & Glennerster H (1990) *Hospital Closure: A political and economic study*. Milton Keynes: Open University Press.

giving an account of the needs assessment of residents both before and five years after resettlement.[24] Our findings revealed that the frequency of psychiatric diagnoses and behaviour problems of those residents from our district resettled in the community from Darenth Park remained fairly consistent. However, the utilisation of local health service provisions, particularly medical outpatients' services, was increased. Similar results were found after a year of the resettlement.[25] In a detailed study carried out on a large sample of resettled Darenth Park residents, Lorna Wing and her colleagues showed no positive outcomes relating to skills improvement and behaviour problems of the resettled residents.[26]

Grove Park Hospital

Grove Park Hospital originally opened as a workhouse in 1908 and in 1919 became a hospital for tuberculosis (TB) patients living in South London. It remained a TB and chest hospital until 1977, when it was redesignated as a facility for people with ID. It had 168 beds, with most of the residents having been transferred from Darenth Park in 1978 following the publication of the white paper *Better Services for the Mentally Handicapped*. In other words, instead of developing community services, a large institution was replaced by a small one! Within a few months after taking up

24 Kon Y & Bouras N (1997) Psychiatric follow-up and health services utilisation for people with learning disabilities. *British Journal of Developmental Disabilities* **84** (1) 20–26.

25 Bouras N, Kon Y & Drummond C (1993) Medical and psychiatric needs of adults with a mental handicap. *Journal of Intellectual Disability Research* **37** (2) 177–182.

26 Wing L (1989) *Hospital Closure and the Resettlement of Residents: The case of Darenth Park Mental Hospital*. Avebury, Aldershot: Gower Publishing Ltd.

my post as consultant psychiatrist I became involved
with Grove Park Hospital, the second long-stay hospital
in our district. I had no contractual obligation to do
so but it was unavoidable; this place needed serious
reforms and preparation for closure after the closure of
Darenth Park.

Of the 168 residents in Grove Park, 99 were the
responsibility of Lewisham and the others of Bromley
district. The process of closing Grove Park was a long one
and took us several years. We had acquired experience
from the closure of Darenth Park, but there were serious
funding problems as the region had limited the funding
to a 'per head basis' and therefore did not allow extra
funding for the special needs of some of the residents.
At that time the Housing Corporation changed its policy
and stopped providing funding for the closure of long-stay
hospitals. The consultant psychiatrist at Grove Park,
Dr Peter Woolf, who had a child psychiatry background
and took a traditional approach to broad medical care in
long-stay institutions for people with ID. He was sceptical
that one day the people living at Darenth Park and Grove
Park could live outside these institutions in community
houses. He was, however, an experienced clinician who
knew the issues involved with long-term institutions.
He retired from the NHS in 1985 and by default I became
the sole consultant psychiatrist responsible for Grove
Park Hospital.

One of our first tasks was to carry out a survey of
all the residents by using the Multi-axial Information
Rating Profile. This is an instrument we developed,
recording social and demographic characteristics, family
history, medical history, a skills assessment scale (for
mobility, sensory, self-help, continence, communication,
literacy and community living), behaviour problems,
a psychopathology scale and service needs. The
difference from the scale used by Lorna Wing in her

research at Darenth Park was that we also measured psychopathology and assessed service needs. The main findings of this survey at Grove Park showed that there was a high incidence of disturbed behaviour; 15% showed depressive features but only 5% were assessed as having symptoms of a psychotic nature. The staff thought that 23% of the residents could live independently, while 41% would need full-time support. We were fortunate that we had developed links with the NUPRD (see also Chapter 2), which published the findings of this survey in a special report.[27]

Intense planning for the closure took place over several years. Emphasis was given to assessing the individual needs of each resident based on the process of 'planning individual needs' (PIN), which was organised, coordinated and executed very thoroughly and systematically by Tracey Power. Regular staff training also took place. The residents were gradually arranged into groups of four to six people with similar needs, in preparation for their resettlement in the community houses. We formally discharged all the residents from psychiatry while they were still at Grove Park Hospital and they were registered with three local GPs. The GPs were employed by Grove Park as clinical assistants and took over the medical care of the residents while we maintained psychiatric involvement as and when necessary.

27 Matt Laws, psychology assistant at the time, led this project very methodically; he was assisted by Vicky Turk, clinical psychologist, and by the psychiatric trainees David Brooks and Katie Drummond who were placed with us at that time. Other psychiatric trainees who worked at Grove Park over the years and contributed to the work included Adrian James, Derek Blincow, Emma Stirland, Chris Cook, Phil Timms, Anne Boucherat and Richard Onaeyo. All of them went on to have a distinguished career in psychiatry. Adrian James became registrar of the Royal College of Psychiatrists; Chris Cook became a professor of psychiatry and Phil Timms became a leading psychiatrist for the mental health problems of homeless people.

Grove Park Hospital closed in 1994 as part of the regional health authority's hospital closure programme, and all the Lewisham residents were resettled into local community-based supported houses. Residents of Bromley were transferred to Bassets, a compound of different sized houses led by consultant psychiatrist Dr Rosalind Bates. The Bromley model of resettlement was different from that of Lewisham. With the closure of Grove Park Hospital there were no longer any long-stay hospital beds for people with ID in the South East Thames Regional Health Authority. It took us 12 years from the start of the Project Group at Guy's to fulfil the main aim of the programme: the resettlement of all the residents from our districts' long-stay institutions into the community.

Chapter 6:
Policy context

Over the period covered in this book, many policy changes occurred that had a direct impact on the services for people with ID. The changing terminology used to refer to people with ID is very noticeable in this chapter; the terms that originally appeared in official documents have been maintained, but intellectual disability (ID) is used in all other circumstances.

As mentioned in the introduction, when I first started working in this field, mental handicap was the term used in the UK and mental retardation in the US. Then the term changed to learning difficulties and then learning disabilities in the UK, while in the US and the rest of the world it became developmental disabilities and then intellectual disabilities. Intellectual disabilities or intellectual disability have now also been adopted in the UK, while the new classification systems are likely to introduce new terms such as 'intellectual developmental disorder'. Only policies and local service developments, structures and restructures that are considered relevant to my work are briefly presented in this chapter. These policies are related to the NHS overall, to mental health specifically and to mental handicap/learning disabilities/intellectual disabilities. New policies were usually followed by local reforms of services, which are briefly described here to help the reader understand the policy context of working as a psychiatrist in London for over 40 years. I have also tried to offer insight into how it felt on a personal level to be involved with many policy changes and at the front line of implementing them.

The main NHS policies that affected the delivery of services for people with mental health and ID included the 1981 white paper *Care in the Community,* which re-emphasised the government's commitment to community care and mandated the closure of long-stay hospitals; the reorganisation of the NHS in 1982, which abolished the area health authorities; the Griffiths Report in 1983, an inquiry into NHS management; and the Mental Health Act (1983), which legislated for the detention of people deemed to be mentally ill and a risk to themselves or others, with or without their consent. The Mental Health Act (1983) included a controversial clause applicable to people with mental handicap, allowing them to be detained because of their disability, and this sparked an ongoing debate.

An influential document was *Reflections on the Management of the National Health Service*, produced in 1985 by the American Professor Alain Enthoven for the Nuffield Trust, and which contributed to the NHS reform programme that followed. In 1989 the then Secretary of State for Health, Kenneth Clark, introduced the white paper, *Working for Patients*, which proposed a split between purchasers and providers of care, GP fund holders and a state-financed internal market, in order to drive service efficiency. These policies were legislated with the National Health Service and Community Care Act (1990). In 1991 the white paper *Health of the Nation* identified a number of important areas for improving health, including cancer, coronary heart disease, mental health and HIV/AIDS.

In 1992 the Tomlinson Report into London's health services created major political conflict about the future of hospitals. That had a direct effect on Guy's Hospital, which lost its accident and emergency department and became 'secondary' to St Thomas' Hospital following a long and contentious debate. In 1994 the number of regional health authorities was reduced to eight.

In 1997 Labour came to power and published the white paper *The New NHS: Modern, dependable*, while in 1999 GP fundholding was abolished and new primary care groups (PCGs) were established. This was followed by *The NHS Plan: A 10-year modernisation programme of investment and reform* in 2000, and in 2002 district health authorities were replaced by strategic health authorities (SHAs) and primary care trusts (PCTs). The National Health Service Reform and Health Care Professions Act (2002) legislated for the redistribution of power from regional health authorities to strategic health authorities. In 2003 the Health and Social Care (Community Health and Standards) Act came into effect. The following year, the first 10 foundation trusts (FTs) were established. These had greater control over their budgets and services. SHAs were reduced from 28 to 10 and the number of PCTs fell from 303 to 152.

Policies that had important direct effects on services for people with ID included the white paper *Better Services for the Mentally Handicapped* in 1971, already referred to in previous chapters, and the *Jay Committee Report* in 1979, in which the influence of normalisation theory was clear, and which set out broad principles relating to the rights of people with mental handicap as well as the principles that should govern service developments.[28] Together with *An Ordinary Life*, published by the Kings Fund in 1980, the Jay

---

28 Rodgers JS (1979) Care of the mentally handicapped: the Jay Committee report. *Lancet* **1** (8120) 816–817.

Committee recommendations represented major policy attempts to reform the services for people with ID.

There was a slow reduction in hospitals in spite of the pressure for change arising from influential policies and the normalisation theory principles, as well as *An Ordinary Life*, which advocated a model of residential care based on ordinary housing. The formation of a pressure group known as ResCare represented a different opinion, by proposing a halt to hospital closures and the creation of village communities. During the late eighties the debate swung firmly towards community care and the eventual closure of the hospitals seemed inevitable. In 1988 'The Griffiths Report', *Community Care: Agenda for action*, intended to sort out the problems between health and social services. This included the long-term or continuing care of dependent groups such as older people, the disabled and the mentally ill. Griffiths stated that community care was not working because no one wanted to accept responsibility for continuing care. *Community Care: Agenda for action* made key recommendations and emphasised that local authorities should have the key role in community care, so social services departments rather than health services should have responsibility for long-term and continuing care, with health services taking responsibility for primary and acute healthcare. This report also specified that social service departments should carry out assessments of care needs in the locality – and set up mechanisms to do this for individuals – and design 'flexible packages of care' to meet these needs. In addition, the Griffiths Report promoted the use of the independent sector. This was to be achieved by social work departments collaborating with and making maximum use of the voluntary and private sources of welfare. Social services should become responsible for registration and inspection of all residential homes, whether run by private organisations or the local authority.

In 1989 the government published its response to the Griffiths Report, the white paper *Caring for People: Community care in the next decade and beyond*. This was a companion paper to *Working for Patients* and shared the same general principles that state provision was bureaucratic and inefficient and that the state should be an 'enabler' rather than a provider of care. The UK state at this time was actually funding, providing and purchasing care for the population, and the separation of the purchaser/provider roles was introduced together with the devolution of budgets and budgetary control. The eighties saw a large expansion of private residential provision, which exceeded the growth in local authority residential provision.

In the 1980s several influential reports with significant policy implications for people with ID were published by the King's Fund Centre, led by Joan Rush and David Towell. One of these was the 1983 publication *Issues and Strategies for Training Staff for Community Services for People with Mental Handicap*, which was based on a series of multidisciplinary workshops that aimed to improve the competencies of staff in community services.[29] Others regularly involved with the King's Fund 'Ordinary Life' activities at that time included Roger Blunden, director of the Mental Handicap Applied Research Unit in Wales, and Richard Brazil of Hummingbird Housing Association. The psychiatrists involved with the King's Fund Centre initiatives at that time included Dr Oliver Russell from Bristol and Dr Mary Myers from Sheffield. Having acquired experience

---

29 Shearer A (ed) (1983) *An Ordinary Life: Issues and strategies for training staff for community services for people with mental handicap*. King's Fund project paper 42. London: King's Fund Centre.

of setting up community services, my colleagues and I were frequently invited to the King's Fund Centre to contribute to its activities, which were very helpful in promoting the principles of community care and the development of quality standards for services.

It should be recognised that the needs and rights of people with ID were brought into focus in the nineties with the growth of advocacy, in particular, citizen advocacy, where a person without ID makes a commitment to advocate for the interests of someone with ID. Advocacy was another significant contributing factor for community care and by the mid-nineties many long stay hospitals had been closed.

Challenging behaviour

While plans and developments for new community-based services were implemented across the country, issues related to people with 'disturbed behaviours' and ID were becoming profound and required practical answers compatible with the philosophy of the new services. In 1986 the King's Fund convened a series of workshops led by Roger Blunden, with the participation of eminent psychologists including Eric Emerson, John Clements, Sandy Toogood, Peter Allen and others, as well as senior managers. Geraldine Holt and I were the psychiatrists invited to participate in this process, together with Mary Myers. Mary made a presentation on the causes of psychiatric problems that might be associated with 'disturbed behaviour' in people with ID and the available treatments. The working group focused on those concepts related to disturbed behaviour in people with ID that could have management implications, under which was subsumed responsibility, accountability, Mental Health Act guidelines and the development of new management policies. Emphasis was given to understanding the reasons for the emergence of 'challenging behaviour', individual planning, and protection of individual rights, communication, occupation, physical environment and staff support.

The term 'challenging behaviour' emerged from these workshops and was defined by Eric Emerson as 'culturally abnormal behaviour(s) of such intensity, frequency or duration that the physical safety of the person or others is placed in serious jeopardy, or behaviour which is likely to seriously limit or deny access to the use of ordinary community facilities'. The importance of the new definition was the conceptual shift from the individual to services and the environment – which were challenged.[30] The term challenging behaviour was gradually widely adopted and replaced the previously used term 'disturbed behaviour'. Challenging behaviour was a social construct not included in any of the diagnostic classification systems and implied that the behaviour of a person with ID challenges the services to rise to meet his/her needs. Many people with ID have challenging behaviour without having an underlying psychiatric diagnosis, while in other cases challenging behaviour and psychiatric disorder may coexist; thus the behaviour may be related to environmental factors alone or to an underlying psychiatric disorder. People with challenging behaviour (in the absence of a psychiatric disorder) are most likely to have severe/moderate ID and have this behaviour due to the contribution of a set of circumstances including poor environment and communication difficulties. Challenging behaviours

30 Blunden R & Allen D (1987) *Facing the Challenge: An ordinary life for people with learning difficulties and challenging behaviour*. King's Fund project paper 74. London: King's Fund Centre.

might be learned by the individual in response to inappropriate staff (carer)actions towards them.

The interface between challenging behaviour and psychiatric disorders has been debated since the time of that King's Fund initiative to today. Several studies, including some of ours, have shown that challenging behaviour can be associated with higher levels of psychiatric disorders.[31] Some polarised views have occurred from time to time, leading to either an underplaying of the links between psychiatric disorders and challenging behaviour or conversely to the overstating of them. A widely held view is that the two interact in complex ways. Professor Anna Cooper has rightly stated that 'the interface between problem behaviours and other mental disorders remain poorly understood, as highlighted by current classificatory manuals for mental disorders. This is despite their common occurence, and that they are distressing for the individual, and can have wider ramifications for the individual and their family and carers.'[32] The distinction between challenging behaviour and mental illness remains one of the key issues and tensions in ID with major clinical and service implications, and unfortunately sometimes becomes the basis of professional rivalries. Colin Hemmings states:

'Some of this is probably driven by lingering anti-medical attitudes and the stigma of mental

31 Hemmings C, Deb S, Chaplin E, Hardy S, Mukherjee R (2013) Review of research for people with intellectual disabilities and mental health problems: A view from the United Kingdom. *Journal of Mental Health Reserach in Intellectual Disability* **6** (2) 127–158.

32 Cooper S-A (2016) Problem behaviours and the interface with psychiatric disorders. In: C Hemmigs and N Bouras (eds) *Psychiatric and Behavioural Disorders in Intellectual and Developmental Disabilities* (3rd edition).Cambridge: Cambridge University Press.

illness by association. Perhaps motivated by the harm caused by lazy labelling and poor quality mental health care some still try to deny the extent of dual diagnosis. Unfortunately this only lets down people with ID. There has been research that appears at least partly motivated by an intention to prove that medication is mostly harmful and ineffective for people with ID. It is difficult to accept this not least because of the low-powered and methodological gaps of existing studies. The truth is that it will always be impossible to neatly separate out mental health problems and challenging behaviour in people with ID. The need for a bio-psychosocial approach, with co-ordinated multidisciplinary input, is arguably nowhere greater in the whole of health care than for people with ID and mental health problems. But very often concurrent trends are contradictory; for example, the desirability of holistic practice or care exists widely in staff or carers' minds whilst there is a concurrent process in services towards more and more super-specialization. Various ways of understanding such as the 'medical' or 'behavioural' or other 'models' are different aids that should be applied simultaneously to provide insights at different levels of mental health problems. Recent research has included statistical approaches to better understand this interface, and started to suggest that there may be a role for the development of emotional regulation strategies. In time, we may be better equipped to assist people with this need.'[33]

33 Hemmings C. & Bouras N (eds) (2016) *Psychiatric and Behavioural Disorders in Intellectual and Developmental Disabilities* (3rd edition). Cambridge: Cambridge University Press.

The controversy and polarised views have had detrimental effects on the development of appropriate services. The situation has led to services mostly overlooking the psychiatric aspects with adverse concequences for service users, their families and carers.

In 1989 the DoH published the report *Needs and Responses: Services for adults with mental handicap who are mentally ill, who have behaviour problems or who offend*.[34] This report was written by a group of psychiatrists specialising in ID and senior managers, who had visited long-stay hospitals, had talked to members of staff as well as to families and carers of people with ID. This report 'reiterated the Government's commitment to community care for people with ID and set as a service objective that by 1991 every district should have policy statements and action plans, agreed with statutory and other agencies concerned, for the care of people with ID, including those who were mentally ill, had behaviour problems or offended'. This report recommended coordinated planning in order to provide comprehensive and integrated services for those with the additional needs of mental illness, behavioural problems and offences. The necessary specialised services could be provided locally, but some of them could be developed on a supra district or regional basis. This was a well thought out and written report that made pragmatic recommendations for the development of the required specialist mental health services for people with ID but was over shadowed by the Mansell Report.

34 Department of Health (1989) *Needs and Responses: Services for adults with mental handicap who are mentally ill, who have behaviour problems or who offend*. London: HMSO.

The Mansell Report

The Mansell Report, commissioned by the DHSS and published in 1993, became one of the most influential policy documents for services for people with ID. The architect was Jim Mansell, professor of psychology at the Tizard Centre at the University of Kent.[35] He was a charismatic personality, a brilliant speaker and a prolific researcher who acquired a high reputation nationally and internationally. He was also very committed to the closure of institutions and the development of community-based services. Members of the working group for the report included Tony Holland, consultant psychiatrist, and Kay Beaumont, social worker, both from the MIETS Unit (see also Chapter 5).

The Mansell Report replaced the terms 'mental handicap' and 'learning difficulties' with 'learning disabilities' (LD), which would be used in the UK. Tony Holland said that it was his idea to introduce the term learning disabilities, as learning difficulties was a very unsatisfactory term. It is fully understandable that service users and families were not happy with the term mental handicap because of the historical stigma attached to it, but I didn't think that 'learning disabilities' was satisfactory either, as I didn't believe it was representative of the issues involved with this population. Learning disabilities was only used in the UK, as in the US and the rest of the world the term mental retardation continued to be used. In addition, the term learning disabilities created confusion with the classification systems in education, where LD referred to learning problems in children who had difficulties with reading, writing and mathematics.

---

35 Department of Health (1993) *Services for People with Learning Disabilities and Challenging Behaviour or Mental Health Needs* (The Mansell Report). London: HMSO.

The terminology continues to be a contentious problem even today, and the debate about the classification of ID and whether to use the term 'disability' or 'disabilities' will probably continue for many years to come.[36]

The key recommendations of the Mansell Report were crucial to developing and sustaining quality services for people with ID to meet local needs. These recommendations provided directions to plan strategically, develop preventative strategies that would avoid crises and to make the most effective use of available funding. The recommendations gave importance to developing and expanding the capacity of local services for people with ID 'to understand and respond to challenging behaviour and to provide specialist services locally which can support good generic practice as well as directly serve a small number of people with the most challenging needs'. There were also several other important recommendations for commissioners, in relation to the development of individualised services and support for families. Additional specialist multidisciplinary support teams for people with challenging behaviour were recommended as an essential component of modern provision. These specialist services needed to use their skills to help managers lead their staff in the provision of effective local services. A closer coordination between the commissioners paying for services, the managers and the professional specialists advising on the support needed by people with ID was necessary to ensure that advice was both practicable and acted upon.

The Mansell Report included very little specifically on mental health services and only stated that

---

36 Bertelli M, Salvador–Carulla L & Harris J (2016) Classification and diagnosis. In: C Hemmings and N Bouras (eds) *Psychiatric and Behavioural Disorders in Intellectual and Developmental Disabilities* (3rd edition). Cambridge: Cambridge University Press.

community-based services should expect generic mental health services to meet the needs of people with ID. This depended on the willingness of mental health services to increase their capacity to work with a new group of patients and the degree of integration of psychiatrists in ID with general psychiatrists. The report continues by stating that 'the appropriate role for psychiatric hospital services for people with ID lay in short-term, highly focused assessment and treatment of mental illness. This implies a small service offering very specifically, closely defined, time-limited services'. That recommendation corresponded to the service provided by MIETS (see also Chapter 5).

The Mansell report was inspirational and thorough. It provided recommendations for people with ID and challenging behaviour, which by that time had become a major problem in the provision and delivery of services. By including mental health/psychiatric needs however, it also created a lot of confusion because of the conceptual differences between mental health needs and challenging behaviour and the required different therapeutic interventions. There was strong criticism of the Mansell Report at the meeting of the Section of Psychiatry in Mental Handicap of the Royal College of Psychiatrists, at their annual meeting in Cambridge in 1993. The criticisms of the Mansell Report were justified and furthermore, the focus on generic mental health services to respond to mental health problems of people with ID was unrealistic. Generic psychiatric services were not prepared to accept people with ID. Most people with ID had more complex mental health needs than those of people without ID who were cared for in generic mental health services. There were also serious funding implications, as generic mental health services received no funding from the closure of the ID institutions because the money was distributed mostly for developing a social care model. The recommendations were interpreted by several commissioners as meaning that they had to focus on services for those with challenging behaviour and overlook those with mental health problems, expecting the generic psychiatric services to meet these needs. In many regions, this policy resulted in people with ID being sent out of their local area to private facilities. Even in our district, where we were developing specialist mental health service for people with ID and were integrated organisationally and managerially with generic mental health services, we experienced serious problems with the commissioners (see also Chapters 8 and 9).

Jim Mansell belonged to a group of psychologists with a profound habitual scepticism about mental illness and psychiatry. We collaborated amicably on several occasions but he never talked about mental health or psychiatry without shifting the emphasis to challenging behaviour and bypassing the differences between the two conditions. Several other prominent psychologists in the UK had a similar attitude to psychiatry, but there were others who were more positive, including the majority of psychology colleagues in the field of ID in the US, Canada and Australia.

In view of the perplexity around specialist mental health services for people with ID that was created by the publication of the Mansell Report, the Department of Health had to issue a clarification note a few months later in June 1994. It was authored by John Garlick, assistant secretary of the Health Care Administration and Peter Bourdillon, senior principal medical officer, and it stated that:

> *'... some authorities had misinterpreted the use of the terms mainstream and generic in the Mansell Report to mean that adults with ID do not require specialist services. Questions had been raised about*

whether to design services which include specialists in the Psychiatry of ID. The Mansell Report does not in fact suggest that specialist mental health services for people with ID are no longer needed. The guidance of the Department of Health makes clear that whilst general NHS services should be used whenever possible, some specialist provision, including specialist mental health services, is also needed. The Mansell Report further emphasised the need to open up generic mental health services to some adults with learning disabilities and reduce the gap which existed between many learning disabilities and mental health services particularly in their organisation.'

Other key policy reports

In 1998 the Department of Health published *Signposts for Success*, an executive document written mostly by Dr Mary Lindsey, past president of the Section of Learning Disability of the Royal College of Psychiatrists and policy advisor at the time. It was the result of an extensive consultation with people with ID, carers and professionals, and aimed to inform on good practice. The main points of the report were that:

'Good practice should rely on such issues as shared values and responsibilities, good quality information and effective training and development. Good practice also should ensure respect of the rights of people with ID, encouraging the use of personal health records, and offering guidance and showing commitment to quality improvement. In general health services, people with ID must have equal rights of access to flexible and responsive services,

*such as specialised dental clinics. Specialist health
services for children and their families, for people
with epilepsy and for people with both learning and
physical or sensory disabilities were all outlined.'*

In 1999 the government launched the National Service
Framework for Mental Health (NSF), which was
the first comprehensive document describing how
mental health services would be planned, delivered
and monitored for the next decade.[37] The NSF did
not mention at all the mental health services for
people with ID, in spite of my suggestion to Graham
Thornicroft, who chaired the working group, that if
they were not addressing people with ID this should
be clearly stated. The rationale for not having such
a statement included in the NSF was that it might
have resulted in pressure to produce a separate policy
document addressing the mental health problems of
people with ID.

Valuing People

In 2001 the white paper *Valuing People* set out how
the government would provide new opportunities
for children and adults with ID and their families to
live full and independent lives as part of their local
communities.[38] This was a very influential inspirational
policy document for people with ID, their families and
carers. The four key principles of *Valuing People* were
rights, independence, choice and inclusion. Soon after
the publication of *Valuing People*, the NHS Executive

---

37 Thornicroft G (1999) *National Service Framework for Mental
    Health*. London: Department of Health.

38 Department of Health (2001) *Valuing People: A new strategy for
    learning disability for the 21st century*. London: Department of
    Health.

and Social Service Inspectorate in London released the report *From Words Into Action*, which outlined the implications of *Valuing People* for the mental health of people with ID. It stated:

'There will be an agreement between ID and mental health services covering all aspects of mental health provision for people with ID. The National Service Framework for Mental Health will apply to services for people with ID who have mental health problems, including the Care Programme Approach (CPA). If a person with ID needs to be treated as an inpatient, they will be admitted to an acute mental health ward. The staff will be competent in supporting people with ID. There will be an agreed approach to emergency admissions. On the rare occasion when acute inpatient wards are not appropriate, people will be treated in small services specifically designed for people with ID, but managed within mental health services. These will serve a number of boroughs. These will probably also provide assessment and treatment services for people with challenging needs. Good local services require very few beds. By 2006, ID and mental health services will have built up competence in local services. A measure of this will be the low use of assessment and treatment beds, combined with a low use of out of borough services and lower usage of psycho-tropic medication. Through the agreement local services will ensure there is provision for mental health services for people with ID and people who have Asperger's Syndrome. The agreement will cover joint working for people with ID who have drug and alcohol problems, eating disorders and other specialist types of mental health need. It will

include the funding responsibilities of ID and mental health services; this will mean that nobody waits whilst funding is resolved. There will be counselling and appropriate therapy available for people with less severe mental health problems. There will be collaborative commissioning on a London wide and a sector basis. Some of these services will fall within the national specialist commissioning remit, when this is agreed. There will be collaborative commissioning for: 'medium secure assessment and treatment services, forensic outreach services,' long term medium secure residential services and semi secure environments and specialist forensic treatments....'

It is obvious that in relation to mental health problems for people with ID, this was a well-intended policy of 'good wishes' making entirely arbitrary recommendations and setting time limits that were not based on any evidence!

Chapter 7: Community mental handicap team

The closure of Darenth Park Hospital (see also Chapter 5) was implemented with the resettlement of the residents from our district to community supported houses. We worked mostly in Lewisham with Providence Partnership and in Southwark with Southwark Consortium. Providence Partnership was a joint venture between Providence Housing Association and Lewisham Mencap. Southwark Consortium for People with Learning Difficulties was established in 1984, as a federation of statutory and voluntary agencies, to develop the supported-housing service for people who had lived in Darenth Park, and to foster the development of a set of comprehensive and coordinated local services for this population. By 1990 it was managing 27 housing projects scattered throughout Southwark, which together housed 150 people with learning difficulties.

The development of the Community Mental Handicap Team (CMHT) was our district's main response to the need for community-based services for people with ID who had been resettled from the institutions, as well as for those living with their families or in social services residential facilities. The CMHT was later renamed the Community Learning Disabilities Team, following the usual trend of renaming. For clarity, I have consistently used the term CMHT in this chapter, because it was used in policy documents at that time. The idea of the CMHT was introduced by Dr Gerald Simon, consultant psychiatrist in Birmingham, founder of the British Institute of Mental Handicap (now BILD) and the first director of the National Development Team in 1981. The National Development Team was set up by the minister Barbara Castle at the Department of Health in the mid-seventies, to facilitate the closure of the long-stay institutions and promote community care for people with ID. Gerald Simon envisioned the CMHT as led by a consultant psychiatrist as a part-time member of staff, with only the nurse and the social worker as full-time members. It was conceived as health service-led and as a method of coordinating service delivery (for example, maintaining close links with all relevant services, developing a close working relationship with child health services, keeping a mental handicap register), providing direct services (for example, making specialist expertise available for people with mental handicap, and providing direct advice, services and support to their families), and as serving a gatekeeper function (for example, making potential services users aware of the range of available services and referring them on). This type of community model with a wide range of functions was very different to the community mental health team described in Chapter 2. The difference between the two types of community team had significant implications for the delivery of mental health service for people with ID. The CMHT had a very heterogeneous multi-professional composition and a very distinct function in service developments, as it was initially concerned with resettlement from the long-stay institutions. The role of the psychiatrist in the newly developed CMHT was unclear; it involved a process of bargaining and negotiation between the members of the team and their respective employers, about roles, orientation and emphasis in this service model.

Within two years, we had established three CMHTs in Lewisham that were coterminous with social services. These CMHTs were for the Northern and Central, Eastern and Southern, and Western and South Western districts. A fourth CMHT was established for the North Southwark area. At this time, trainee psychiatrists from the Guy's psychiatric training scheme rotated every six months into our service. This was a great help to me, as for the first two years I was working single-handedly, with increasing clinical demands as well as organisational and service developments.[39]

The core membership of each of the CMHTs included a patch manager, support manager, patch administrator, clinical psychologist, occupational therapist, physiotherapist, speech therapist, social worker and psychiatrist. This was an impressive mix of professionals and managers, but some had no knowledge of mental health problems, and furthermore, had several other roles related to skills development and supports for people with ID.[40] A great deal of work was generated by the closure of Darenth Park, such as the development of residential community houses, furnishing them, organising the support staff as well coordinating the liaison with other relevant health and social services. I had to attend an excess of meetings every day, but only a handful of them were relevant to psychiatry. While several colleagues were

---

39 The first psychiatric trainee was David Brooks, followed by Katie Drummond. Both became consultant psychiatrists in ID. David Brooks remained in the group of core colleagues of consultant psychiatrists in ID at Bexley and later Lambeth until he moved outside London in 2004. After completing her training with us Katie Drummond joined St George's Hospital and Medical School.

40 We enjoyed from the beginning the benefit of an impressive team of clinical psychologists, including Catherine Dooley, Vicky Turk, Theresa Joyce, Sheena Henney, Anna Eliatamby, Andrea Hughes, Avril Missen, Barley Oliver and others.

supportive of the new developing role of the psychiatrist, including the director of services Nan Karl, there were others who were aversive or even antagonistic. It was not on a personal level, but nevertheless, this attitude was annoying and frustrating, and affected the psychiatric trainees, who found it difficult to accept.

At the operational level, there were problems with general psychiatry colleagues who were either asking me to take over existing service users with a degree of ID, or refusing to accept new cases. The situation was worse if admission was required as there were no inpatient beds available for the admission of people with ID anywhere in the district. It was obvious to me that the CMHT model, with such a diverse synthesis of professionals delivering multi-heterogeneous tasks, was not the right model of community service for the mental health provision of people with ID. After the responsibility of having to provide care for some of the resettled people with complex needs from Darenth Park and Grove Park, and new referrals coming through from general psychiatry and GPs, service users living independently or with their parents and families daunted me. I came to believe that the delivery of mental health care from a CMHT was a historical mistake because it transferred into the community an institutional model of care. Eddie Chaplin referred to this model as a 'one stop shop', just as it was in the institutions.[41]

The operational policy of the CMHT in our service stated: 'The CMHT is the mechanism through which within each patch the range of skills and services available to support service users are brought together in order to review the way in which services are being

41 Chaplin E, Paschos D, O'Hara J, McCarthy J, Holt G, Bouras N & Tsalanikos E (2010) Mental ill-health and care pathways in adults with intellectual disability across different residential types. *Research in Developmental Disabilities* **31** (2) 458–463.

delivered and identify ways in which the service
can be improved.' This was a valuable definition but
lacked any specifics for delivering a mental health
service. I then defined the role of the psychiatrist in
the CMHT as having clinical involvement with clinical
responsibility and also a consultative role. The clinical
responsibilities included mental health assessment,
treatment of diagnosable psychiatric disorders,
monitoring psychotropic medication, contributing to the
management of epilepsy and liaison with other medical
doctors as appropriate. The consultative role included
contribution to the management of behaviour problems
in a multidisciplinary forum, and providing support to
relatives and care staff.

In 1988 Rob Greig took over as director of our service.[42]
Rob Greig was a dynamic and inspiring manager with
strong views, who after leaving our service became a
visible figure in ID services, holding senior positions
including, among others, the government's National
Director for Learning Disabilities and the main author of
the policy document *Valuing People* (see also Chapter 6).
He took over the management of our service at the peak
of the developments, at which point there were several
services up and running (including supported houses), the
commitment to close Grove Park, and close interaction
with social services.

Within the framework of important structural
changes that were taking place in the 1980s and 1990s
in the NHS (see also Chapter 6), Rob Greig focused his
energy on the organisation of services, the continuation
of the planned reforms and the strengthening of the

---

42 He replaced Nan Karl, who left for King's Fund College where
she developed a programme on leadership. Rob Greig had been
working in a junior administrative position with Elaine Murphy,
professor of psychiatry of old age at Guy's, who also became
district general manager for Lewisham and North Southwark
Health Authority from 1984 until 1990.

community presence of people with ID, within the
financial constraints of that time. He oversaw the
closure of Grove Park Hospital at a very difficult
financial time, when funding for the closure of long-
stay hospitals was not forthcoming. He had an overt
ambiguity in his decisions relating to psychiatry, where
his lack of clarity and a certain degree of habitual
scepticism posed difficulties. He failed to appreciate
the specialist role of mental health service in ID and
the problems involved in trying to deliver clinical care
from a multidisciplinary heterogeneous CMHT, and
was a strong advocate of generic mental health services
without, however, being able to facilitate the interfaces
involved.

Within the CMHT structure, we spent a lot of time
on issues unrelated to a mental health service and that
was raised regularly by trainees who, despite finding
the experience of specialist aspects of mental health
for people with ID rewarding, were perplexed by the
demands imposed on them to sort out non-psychiatric
issues, for example, residential care, benefits, recreation,
etc. The complex issues and fundamental contradictions
in the organisation of CMHTs, which affected them
because of their extensive diversity, were described
by our colleagues Geraldine Holt and Barley Oliver,
in their 1989 article *Reducing Stress in Community
Mental Handicap Teams*.[43]

---

43   Holt G & Oliver B (1989) Reducing stress in community mental
     handicap teams. *Mental Handicap* **17** (1) 4–5.

Chapter 8: Specialist mental health service

Specialist versus mainstream mental health services

There was no doubt in my mind that if the community care plans for people with ID were to have any chance of success, they needed to be supported by a responsive, strong mental health provision. This provision could not be developed either from ID services alone or generic mental health services alone; it needed the support and collaboration of both systems. Furthermore, it became even clearer that the role of the psychiatrist should be to focus on how best to meet the mental health needs of people with ID as well as taking an advisory role in the broader issues of health and social care.

The overall position of governmental policy all along was that people with ID should have access to generic (that is, for anyone, with or without ID) health services, but with additional specialist (specifically for people with ID) support when needed. The argument in favour of generic services providing mental health care for people with ID appeared sound and was supported widely. There was the argument that specialised services lead to stigmatisation, labelling and negative professional attitudes. A counter-argument, however, was that special expertise was required for the diagnosis and treatment of psychiatric disorders in people with ID, because although it is theoretically possible to train staff in generic settings, the relatively small number of cases gives little opportunity for staff to gain or maintain the necessary skills. Problems arise particularly when admissions to generic adult acute inpatient units occur, as people with ID often require longer admissions, and may be vulnerable without additional support on the ward. Furthermore, people with ID represent a very heterogeneous group with a varied range of highly complex mental health needs, which generic staff may be ill-equipped to meet. Services should be provided according to need and delivered in the context of both ID and psychiatric disorders coexisting, in order to allow for more appropriate treatment, support, service planning and development. A partnership between the generic mental health and ID service structures is necessary to ensure responsive support and treatments to previously under-served individuals. Our vision was to provide high quality mental health care to people with ID and mental health needs. We believed that by developing a specialist mental health service in collaboration with generic adult mental health services, together with other necessary supports, we would enable people with ID to live a normal life as much as possible.

We had already started outpatient clinics at psychiatric outpatient departments at the Munro Clinic at Guy's in 1983, Lewisham Hospital in 1984 and in New Cross Gate General Practice Centre the same year. The latter did not last long as it was little used either by service users or the local GPs. It was not easy to gain access to run the outpatient clinics because of the various obstacles imposed by administrators regarding the suitability of their premises for our population, the administrative support and so on.

The real breakthrough for the development of our service came in 1988 with the appointment of the first community psychiatric nurse (CPN) initially appointed euphemistically as a senior clinical support worker. The reason for not using the term CPN was that it was not politically correct at that time to appoint 'nurses' for services supporting people with ID. Paula McAlpine was the first CPN and led the future developments for CPNs, which were successfully expanded later by Mei Jones, until she moved on to Wales, and then by Lynette Kennedy, who eventually became team leader. It should be pointed out that the appointment of the first senior clinical support worker was fully supported and facilitated by Nan Karl, director of services, and Dot Wootton, community manager. Together with the psychiatric trainees who at the time were placed in our service as part of their rotation, David Brooks as senior registrar and Katie Drummond as registrar, we gave an identity to our service. It was a community-based service and we initially called it Assessment Intervention Mental Handicap Service (AIMS) but soon opted for Psychiatry of Mental Handicap Service. We presented its mode of working as an integrated bridge between ID and generic mental health services.

Administratively and operationally, we became autonomous from the CMHTs, with whom we maintained strong functional and operational links for multidisciplinary working. At the same time, we moved our base to the grounds of Grove Park Hospital, where we had access to spacious offices. My base remained at the Guy's academic psychiatry department but I joined colleagues at Grove Park at regular times every week. We also started a series of negotiations with generic adult psychiatry colleagues to acquire two or three inpatient admission beds at the York Clinic at Guy's. Despite lengthy discussions, working and steering groups, and support from senior managers (including Elaine Murphy who was then general district manager) and all the consultant general psychiatrists, we failed to develop this inpatient facility. The only reservation expressed with regards to its development was from Catherine Dooley, top grade psychologist (as the job title was then) in ID, on the grounds that any inpatient admission should have a long-term plan of care attached. Obviously this would have been self-explanatory if we had the admission beds, but we did not have them. The solution was offered by Professor Jim Watson, who was a great inspiration, facilitator and supporter from the start of the service until his retirement. Jim made available to us two inpatient admission beds on Maurice Craig ward, then the professorial inpatient psychiatric unit of the York Clinic at Guy's Hospital. This arrangement worked out well, and allowed us to admit and successfully treat some people with ID and mental health problems. In 1988 we published an article that referred to a difficult case of severe eating disorder in an adult man with Down's syndrome who made a good recovery based on a 'rewards programme' implemented by the ward nurses with our support.[44] Over 10 years after the publication of our article about using a generic psychiatric ward for the admission of people with ID, reports were published by others describing their use of generic psychiatric wards as a 'new, innovative idea'.

We emphasised that our service was 'an integrated mental health service for people with ID'. However, the description of our service as 'integrated' created problems with some colleagues who thought that we were advocating that there was no need for a

44 Holt G, Bouras N & Watson JP (1988) Down's syndrome and eating disorders: A case study. *British Journal of Psychiatry* **152** (6) 847–848.

specialist service. This led to a debate with Dr Ken Day, consultant psychiatrist at Northgate Hospital Morpeth, Northumberland, and strong advocate of specialist psychiatry for people with ID. Ken Day was one of the few psychiatrists who at that time were clear about the role of a psychiatrist in the field of ID. Several other psychiatrists focused on genetic syndromes, epilepsy, and the social and educational aspects of this population. This diversity of opinion, a well-known phenomenon in the NHS, is welcome, but there should be a limit to it diluting the role of psychiatrists and it can become confusing for commissioners and managers.

It is worth noting here the long-standing debate in the Section of Mental Handicap of the Royal College of Psychiatrists about whether or not there should be a 'life span' service or separate services for children and adults. For years, influential colleagues in the Royal College of Psychiatrists advocated strongly a life span service. I always thought that it was a spurious argument, as different competencies were required for children and adults, and there were well-established separate child and adult generic mental health services for those without mental handicap. Dr Sarah Bernard and Professor Jeremy Turk clarified the issues for child learning disabilities services in a very informative publication.[45] Sarah trained at Guy's with us and remained a close colleague over the years. Jeremy worked initially with the St George's service and later moved to the South London and Maudsley Foundation NHS Trust. We collaborated very closely with Jeremy Turk over the years, as well as with his wife, Vicky Turk, senior clinical psychologist at Grove Park Hospital and later consultant psychologist for the ID services of the Oxleas NHS Foundation Trust.

---

45 Bernard S & Turk J (2009) *Developing Mental Health Services for Children and Adolescents: A toolkit for clinicians*. London: Royal College of Psychiatrists.

In an effort to avoid the confusion with 'integrated service', we started using the term 'specialist mental health service'. This created another misunderstanding for some working within ID services, who thought that we were presenting a 'specialist overall ID service', which was an outdated concept and not harmonious with the current philosophy of services. We argued that we were not an overall ID service but equivalent with the other specialist mental health services in the UK, such as those for children and adolescents, older adults, rehabilitation, addictions, eating disorders, women's mental health, and so on.

Faculty of the Royal College of Psychiatrists

In the 1980s the strong ideologies and policies referred to in Chapters 4 and 5 dominated the emerging new services and the role of the psychiatrist in ID became very blurred. The UK is the only country that has trained psychiatrists specialising in the mental health problems of people with ID. This is probably due to the UK's health system, with the NHS providing universal healthcare for the whole population, and to the fact that the Royal College of Psychiatrists has significantly raised the standards of training, contributing to an improvement in the quality of care for people with ID.

The Section of Mental Handicap of the Royal College of Psychiatrists published an important document in 1983, which described the roles and responsibilities of the psychiatrist working and supporting people with ID.[46] Reports were coming in from many parts of the country, however, stating that psychiatrists were marginalised

---

46 Royal College of Psychiatrists (1983) Mental handicap services—
The Future. *Psychiatric Bulletin* **7** (7) 131–134.

and the mental health aspects of people with ID were overlooked during the process of closing the long-stay hospitals and the then dominant emphasis on social care and normalisation theory principles.[47]

In our district we were very fortunate to recruit young psychiatrists to our training scheme, both as part of their general psychiatry training at registrar level and at the higher speciality level of senior registrars in ID. The fact that we were part of the extended rotational general psychiatry training scheme of Guy's was very beneficial. Our higher training in the psychiatry of ID had been reviewed and approved by the Speciality Higher Training Committee of the Royal College of Psychiatrists. An added value for our training scheme, which helped to attract high-calibre trainee colleagues, was the strong links we had developed with the academic psychiatry department at Guy's as part of the UMDS and later King's College London, and our applied health service research activities (see also Chapter 11).[48]

In 1988 Yvonne Wiley, then president of the Section of Mental Handicap of the Royal College of Psychiatrists, invited me to become a member of the Joint Mental Handicap Committee for Higher Training, where I stayed until 1993 when my term expired. I worked very closely with other colleagues, and

---

47 Nwulu BN (1988) Consultant jobs in mental handicap: Dead end posts? *Psychiatric Bulletin* **12** 279–281.

48 Several colleagues were trained in our higher training scheme and became consultant psychiatrists in the field of ID or in joint posts with general psychiatry; among them were David Brooks, Geraldine Holt, Emmanouela Akande, Titi Akinsola, Sarah Bernard, Agnieska Bokzanska, Jackie Conway, Katie Drummond, Annabel Dudley, Mo Eyeoyibo, Peter Hughes, Colin Hemmings, John Gavilan, Shaun Gravestock, Yan Kon, Joanna Mulvey, Brendan McCormack, Elizabeth Obe, Dimitrios Paschos, Max Pickard, Alaa Al-Sheikh, Mathew Stevenson, Clive Timehin, Shahid Zaman, Robert Winterhalder, Hugh Williams, Mike Vanstralem and Kiriakos Xenitidis.

particularly with Dr Jack Piachaud. Together we carried out several review visits – known then as approval visits – around the country, during which we advised on training schemes. This included advising about raising the standards of training and creating posts in our field that would be attractive to new trainees. It was a very interesting experience, full of hope and expectations that with service reforms the standards of care could be raised.

In 1990 I was a member of the Royal College of Psychiatrists' working party on multi-axial classification, which was led by Mrs Jennifer Rohde of the Department of Public Health and Epidemiology of Charing Cross and Westminster Medical School, with Professor Sheila Hollins, Professor Ben Sacks, Dr Jeremy Bird, Dr Val Anness and Maria Callias. We published a report in 1993 that recommended the use of multi-axial classification for people with ID.[49]

In 1992 Jose Jancar and Yvonne Wiley nominated me for honorary secretary of the Section but I was not elected. Instead I was elected as a member of the Executive Committee, where I stayed until 1996 when my term expired. During this time, I served on several committees of the college. I have the greatest respect for Yvonne Wiley. While she was president of the Section we regularly exchanged ideas, and she would often ask my opinion on several service and training issues. The main theme was service developments and raising standards of care. I carried out several commitments for the college, for example, as assessor on advisory appointments committees for consultant posts and as regional advisor. I was also clinical tutor in psychiatry at Guy's from 1991 to 1996 and worked closely with the

---

49 Anness V, Bhat A, Bouras N, Callias M, Hollins S, Rohde J & Sacks B (1991) A multi-aspect assessment for people with mental handicap. *Psychiatric Bulletin* **15** 146.

training scheme organiser Joe Herzberg. Joe Herzberg worked very methodically to systematise the training scheme, which was also expanded to a wider area of the South East Thames Region. A comprehensive handbook and regular assessments of the trainees were introduced by Joe, together with recurring clinical tutors' meetings.

I was a member of the Joint Working Group of the Sections for Psychiatry and General Psychiatry, which produced the first report on *Meeting the Mental Health Needs of Adults with Mild Learning Disabilities* in 1996, with Neill Simpson as convenor and other members Greg O'Brien, Allan Calvert, Adrienne Regan, Desmond Dunleavy and Terry Nelson. The report recommended the development of specialist mental health teams that would ensure coordinated and effective liaison and integration with other agencies. It stated that the teams would need to have expertise in both ID and mental health, and be able to provide a direct service to people with ID and their carers, and training and advice to other agencies. It advised that these teams should be based locally, providing inpatient care and outpatient and community-based interventions.

The name of the Section changed from Mental Handicap to Learning Disabilities in 1993 following a re-run of the first tie-breaker ballot when the term LD had received 84 votes and mental handicap 83 votes. At the re-run LD had 33%, mental handicap 29%, developmental psychiatry 18% and developmental neuropsychiatry 13%.

On several occasions, I wrote to successive presidents of the Section (later renamed the Faculty of Learning Disabilities) and to policy advisors at the Department of Health, to raise various issues about the lack of clarity in policy related to mental health needs of people with

ID. For instance, I wrote in 1997: 'I have represented the College recently in advisory appointments committees in the Greater London area. In all cases I found the job descriptions very unsatisfactory. The role of the Consultant Psychiatrist appeared to be rather an adviser to planning of services than a clinician with identified clinical role and responsibilities. All the posts were for consultants working alone with very few prospects of having junior staff.' In another instance, I wrote in 1999:

'Joint commissioners seem to be apprehensive that the mental health services for people with intellectual disabilities will be under social services management. The concern is that such a possibility would lead to a greater fragmentation of services for people with intellectual disabilities and mental health needs than the current situation. Although this is a local matter it seems to me a paradox that LD-NHS Trusts still retain specialist mental health services, particularly in those areas where there are no long stay NHS residential beds. I believe that the natural place for any mental health service, including for people with intellectual disabilities, would be within the generic mental health services of the local area. There are of course funding implications and I can see the reluctance of generic services to undertake that responsibility unless transference of proper resources is agreed. I also think that it is not appropriate for the mental health needs of people with intellectual disabilities to be included under the title of 'health care', which is usually confused and diluted with all aspects of physical health. With the same logic, the LD-NHS Trusts should have been providing neurological and orthopaedic care etc. I believe that it would be a great

> *mistake if the specialist component of mental health*
> *for people with learning disabilities is locked in*
> *organisational structures of the past or is dominated*
> *by ideological and philosophical views.'*

I was not invited to take any active role in the faculty affairs after 1996, but the colleagues involved raised the visibility of the speciality and contributed to raising the standards of training and recruitment into the speciality. It is unclear what influence the faculty might have had on policy. In 2007 I was invited to join the Board of International Affairs and the editorial board of *International Psychiatry* as editor of special papers.

The local landscape

In the 1990s more national policies, reports and documents were published that profoundly affected both services and people with ID during this decade and the future. Some of them are described in Chapter 6. In this current chapter a brief description is presented of the most important local changes related to the delivery of our services.

In 1989 South East Thames Health Regional Authority reaffirmed the massive shift of emphasis to community-based care, which had been accompanied by major changes in attitudes about how services should be provided to people with learning difficulties.[50] Positive developments in supported residential housing were described, though not with a uniform model of care, and emphasised that new services should be tailored to individual needs and individual programmes should be developed. This report included the important

---

50 SETHRA (1989) *A Review of Policy for People with Learning Difficulties*. London: SETRHA.

statement that, 'once social care services for people with leaning difficulties have been transferred, the role of the NHS would become one of providing health care through the generic health care services of the primary health care team and the district general hospital and other specialised health services. Staff in these services need help to adjust to meeting the needs of citizens who have Learning Difficulties.' This direction was adopted in all subsequent central and local policies and had profound implications for the mental health care of people with ID. The expectation was that generic mental health services would respond by taking over the mental health care of people with ID by skilling up their staff but without being offered any additional resources, because money was tied up with social care (see also Chapter 5). There was very little mention of the 'special needs' of people with ID, and the recommendation to revise the *Mental Handicap Special Services* document produced in 1984 (see also Chapter 6) was never realised.

A significant change at a local level was that Guy's Hospital became an NHS trust in 1990 and three years later merged with St Thomas' Hospital to form the Guy's and St Thomas' Hospital NHS Trust. The Lewisham and Guy's Mental Health NHS Trust was established shortly afterwards, in 1994, following the separation of mental health from acute health services NHS trusts. The first CEO of the Lewisham and Guy's Mental Health NHS Trust was Peter Reading, who had worked as a trainee health service administrator in the early stages of our developments with the AHMT. With Peter's support, we succeeded in moving the management of our specialist mental health service – which now included psychology and 'challenging needs specialists' – from the ID management unit to the generic mental health services structure. This was a major organisational breakthrough because from that time we rightly belonged to the crowd of mental health professionals with whom we shared the same skills and expertise but with a focus on people with ID and mental health problems. Initially, organisationally and managerially, we were under the Adult Mental Health Unit but soon, with the restructuring of the trust, we formed a separate mental health in ID directorate in 1994, with service manager Phil Woods, who was also managing the older adults' mental health directorate. Both Peter Reading and Phil Woods were very supportive and that made a significant contribution to our work. The first clinical director of our new directorate was Theresa Joyce, senior clinical psychologist and later consultant psychologist. Our specialist service was renamed the Mental Health in Learning Disabilities (MHiLD) service. The close collaboration with clinical psychologists at clinical and academic levels further strengthened our service.

However, while there was such important progress operationally, the commissioning of our service remained as complicated and unclear as ever – and this situation followed me up to the date of my retirement! The implementation of the National Health Service and Community Care Act (1990), and the separation of commissioning and provision of services, created an extraordinary confusion for services for people with ID and those with additional mental health needs in our local boroughs of Lewisham and Southwark. The main reasons for this were the distribution of funding attached to institutions after their closure, the different interpretation of the ever-changing regulations by the various commissioners, and the high financial cost of providing a mental health service for people with ID. In some quarters there was also an overt aversion to psychiatry, not on a personal level but as a matter of principle! The funding for our service was hidden from the closure of the institutions in what was called 'health budget'. The 'health budget' covered the cost of the CMHTs, which were expected to provide some mental health care. However, the main bulk of mental health care for people with ID was expected to be provided by generic mental health services, even though they were not offered any additional resources from ID, as mentioned earlier. Generic mental health services argued – rightly, in my opinion – that they were neither commissioned nor had the expertise to meet the mental health needs of people with ID.

In the early 1990s the commissioning of our local mental health services, as well as ID services, was undertaken by the then newly formed South East Commissioning Agency as part of the Priority Care Unit of the South East London Health Authority (SELHA), later to become Lambeth, Southwark and Lewisham Health Commission (known as LSL). The commissioning arrangements for health and social care for people with ID in the three London boroughs of Lambeth, Southwark and Lewisham were different. A decision was made that the generic mental health services and services for people with ID would be borough based, which created problems of disaggregating and separating the existing budgets. This had unavoidably serious repercussions for our service.

Lewisham Partnership was set up in 1992/3 on the initiative of Rob Greig, then director of services in ID (see also Chapter 8). It was established as a management agency with mixed joint commissioning and provider functions, when the priority care unit of Lambeth, Southwark and Lewisham Health Authority (LSL), was divided into Mental Health Trust and Optimum Community Trust. The intention was for Lewisham Partnership to act as a jointly funded independent agency, commissioning residential nonprofit organisations, social care and health services for adults with intellectual disabilities in the borough of Lewisham. This was an innovative, admirable and promising idea that was lost in the implementation, defeated by the lack of clarity in the competing demands of health and social care! Wendy Wallace was appointed as the CEO of the Lewisham Partnership. The management of the CMHTs became unclear, as Lewisham Partnership appeared to function as both commissioner and provider, and tried to bring our management back under the ID management unit. However, we eventually succeeded in remaining under Lewisham and Guy's Mental Health Trust. There were additional serious problems with the commissioning of residential supported houses for those people with ID and additional complex mental health needs, most of whom ended up in placements 'out of area' at major financial expense (see also Chapters 8 and 9).

Optimum Health Care was a community trust that emerged at the same time as Lewisham Partnership. Optimum Health Care was primarily a provider of speech and language therapy, and occupational therapy delivered through the CHMTs, which added to the confusion of the maze that was local NHS organisational structures.

In the borough of Southwark the situation was even more confusing. The commissioners of the Lambeth, Southwark and Lewisham Health Authority (LSL) had different 'pots of money' identified for specific projects for people with ID and these were separate from social services, which were supposed to commission social care. What is classified as a health need, as opposed to a social care need, for people with ID is not always clear and the distinction between the two can be very artificial. Joint commissioning of health and social care for people with ID was implemented in Southwark at the end of

1997 – much later than in Lewisham. The existence of Southwark Consortium in the borough as a provider of mainly, but not only, residential care, complicated the picture even further. Southwark Consortium had a block funding contract with the NHS to provide residential services after the closure of Darenth Park for people with ID who originated from the whole borough of Southwark, while our catchment area was restricted to North Southwark only. Considerable funding was available to Southwark Consortium to commission services from MIETS at Bethlem Royal Hospital at its discretion. There were historically several people from the South Southwark area placed outside the area, at major expense, mostly by social services, some of whom had been residents in Darenth Park. The provision of generic mental health services and ID services for Lambeth and South Southwark was provided then by the Maudsley Hospital. In 1993 Lachlan Campbell, consultant psychiatrist for South Southwark and Lambeth, resigned, releasing his joint post with MIETS Unit at Bethlem Royal Hospital. In the meantime, Tony Holland was appointed to a new ID chair in Cambridge, leaving MIETS without consultant psychiatrist cover. MHiLD service at Guy's stepped in and made an interim arrangement for Dr Shaun Gravestock, who was eligible in the final stages of his training as senior registrar to become acting locum consultant under my supervision, pending a substantive appointment.

With all this perplexity in commissioning services for people with ID, the different providers of specialist services in Southwark they were expressing interest in providing the mental health services, though without any specialist knowledge or expertise in mental health. The main aim was presumably to obtain some additional funding. However, the funding for the mental health of ID in Southwark was held firmly by Lambeth,

Southwark and Lewisham Health Commissioning (LSL), where Doug Adams, the deputy director for mental health, had a good understanding of the complex situation and was trying to protect our specialist service. I should also mention that, reflecting back, I always felt that there was a better understanding of our issues among professionals and managers in generic mental health services than among those in ID services.

It is amazing how all these complexities were allowed to mushroom in the NHS, creating an unbelievable bureaucracy and fragmentation that hampered the delivery of care in a health system admired around the world for providing easy access to services that are free at the point of contact. In my experience of working in the NHS for over 35 years, I believe that the organisational problems were complicated not only by the lack of funding, but equally, if not more so, by the personalities involved. Considering how many problems we experienced in a small service such as ours, I wondered what would happen in other services in the NHS as a whole.

Chapter 9: Mental Health in Learning Disabilities Service

In spite of the turmoil of changes imposed by new policies and organisational contradictions the specialist mental health in ID services expanded due to the acceptance and recognition by service users, families and carers and the dedication and the commitment of colleagues. This happened regardless of the fact that we seemed not to inhabit the same world with some of the commissioners.

By that time we had become known as the Mental Health in Learning Disabilities Service (MHiLD). Our operational policy stated that 'MHiLD is a specialist service as an integral part of mental health services with the aim to meet the mental health needs of adults with ID living in our catchment area', and that 'the service offers specialist assessment, advice and treatment of mental health problems and promotion of mental well-being delivered in partnership with the local multi-disciplinary intellectual disabilities services, psychology and behavioural support services and adults with disabilities social services teams'. MHiLD provided compressive assessment and treatment to adults with ID who displayed evidence of psychiatric illness and/or personality disorder, and those with high-risk behaviour but with no diagnosed mental health problem requiring specialist psychiatric intervention.

More community psychiatric nurses (CPNs) – no longer called senior clinical support workers – were appointed, and we were given much-needed and appreciated administrative support. When Grove Park Hospital closed, we lost our service base there and transferred it to the top floor of the Munro Outpatient Psychiatric Clinic at Guy's. In fact, we literally squatted there, and stayed until our next stage of development! The most difficult problem we faced was the lack of admission beds, as the professorial unit at the York Clinic at Guy's was closed and we lost the access to the two beds we had there. The district generic psychiatric services were undergoing massive restructuring and frequent reorganisation, and they had lost a significant number of acute admission beds. At the same time, the psychiatry admission beds in other parts of the district, at Bexley and Hither Green hospitals, were marked for closure. Without access to the beds at the York Clinic, when an admission was needed we had to negotiate with the psychiatric inpatient service in the catchment area of the service user. This was a difficult and lengthy process, as there were several catchment areas and several acute admission wards in three sites at Guy's, Lewisham and Hither Green Hospitals. Obviously, each ward had different staff, different attitudes and philosophies, and we had to explain again and again the reasons for requesting admission and be interrogated as to why MHiLD did not have admission beds. Furthermore, several of our service users were not fulfilling the tight acute admission criteria of adult psychiatry, and we constantly faced a variety of barriers from generic mental health services that would not accept our requests for admission.

The pressure on our service was enormous, as the

long-stay hospitals had closed, many new community residential services were up and running all over the district and new referrals were coming in from people living with their families. Some of our referrals requiring inpatient admission were certainly not suitable for acute psychiatric wards either, because of the level of their challenging behaviour, their level of disability or other very complex clinical issues. There was no alternative other than to admit them to a private hospital out of area. Then the search for a bed started, but the most difficult problem was identifying funding. Whose responsibility was the cost, which was always expensive, for such cases? MHiLD had no such funding available. Was it the responsibility of generic psychiatric services? Was it the responsibility of the local social services departments? Was it the responsibility of the commissioning health authority? Health service commissioners argued with social services that it was not a health problem for the psychiatric services but an ID problem for social services, and social services counter-argued that it was a health problem. This was exactly as Frank Menolascino had stated in the USA in the 1980s (see also Chapter 4). No one was willing to accept responsibility and at the operational level for the clinical team of MHiLD it was a real nightmare.

These were monumental issues of an NHS fragmented bureaucracy with no one accepting responsibility in spite of so many people being involved, leaving the problem to a powerless clinical team. The common resolution was to have yet another 'working group' or 'steering group' to discuss the problems and the issues, to identify ways of 'joint working' and 'shared values', and to try and prevent these problems occurring again. I participated in endless meetings and working groups of this type, and I have kept masses of notes and archives, all of which demonstrate the same approach of 'passing the parcel' or avoiding the problem!

The problem of lacking local admission inpatient facilities for those people with ID and mental health problems, including some people with challenging behaviour, reached huge proportions when the numbers of people being sent out of their local area to private services started growing noticeably. Some districts made more use of placing people with ID out of area in private services than others. In 2008 it was estimated that in England there was a reduction (24%) in the overall number of inpatients from 4,435 in 2006 to 3,376 in 2010. Within that, the proportion of people with ID, mostly with challenging behaviour and/or mental health problems, in independent sector provision rose from 21% to 32%, and the number of independent sector providers increased from 48 to 61.[51]

In desperation in the face of these problems, MHiLD service worked out a temporary solution. I took over the clinical responsibility of one of the inpatient rehabilitation adult psychiatry wards (T1) of the Lewisham area, in Bexley Hospital, in exchange for being able to admit there those people with ID who were suitable for such inpatient admission. That ward was marked for closure and it was thought that the Bexley Hospital Resettlement Team would benefit from my previous experience of the Darenth Park and Grove Park closures. I had the opportunity to work with excellent nursing staff at the T1 ward in Bexley Hospital, and together with colleagues from MHiLD we developed skills to successfully support those people with ID who had to be admitted there. At the same time, we had a very fruitful collaboration with Isobel Morris, senior clinical psychologist leading the Bexley Hospital re-provision of services in the community plan and Jo Kent, project

51 Emerson E & Robertson J (2008) *Commissioning Person-centred, Cost Effective, Local Support for People with Learning Disabilities.* London: Social Care Institute of Excellence.

manager. The re-provision of services in Bexley had some distinctly different features to the closure of the Darenth and Grove Park hospitals. The most important of these was that for those with special needs, additional supports were built in to their residential accommodation. Bexley Hospital closed eventually and the Lewisham service users were successfully re-provided with community services, but we lost the inpatient access to T1 ward, which had been a significant help.

In the meantime, MHiLD continued to consolidate its position as a specialist mental health service for people with ID across the region. Vacant consultant psychiatrists' posts, following either retirement or the development of new posts, were taken up by those who had completed their training in our rotational scheme. A network of colleagues built up gradually around the neighbouring districts. These were a new breed of consultant psychiatrists who shared the same values around supporting people with mental health needs and ID, and made significant contributions to the development of local services. The links with colleagues in the region were strong, as they became members of the Section of Psychiatry of Mental Handicap, later renamed Psychiatry of ID, which was part of the Division of Psychiatry and Psychology of UMDS. Consultant psychiatrist colleagues were offered an honorary senior lecturer appointment with the Medical School of UMDS and had protected time from their service commitments to contribute to teaching, training, research and development. This was a major strength of our organisations, and one that contributed decisively to the development of services and helped to promote health service research (see also Chapter 11).

Brendan McCormack, at the last part of his higher specialist training, was appointed as acting consultant psychiatrist for the Bexley area in 1988 and stayed there for a year until he moved to Dublin in Ireland to take up a joint post in adult general psychiatry and ID. David Brooks took up the substantive post of consultant psychiatrist in ID for Bexley in 1989 and remained there until 1997 when he moved to Lambeth. David remained very closely involved with us and the Section of UMDS and was one of the main pillars of our organisation. At about the same time, Dr Sabah Sadik moved from Liverpool to a new joint post with the Section of UMDS at Medway, following lengthy negotiations for the development of this post with Helen Mair, regional public health physician and strong supporter of the development of high-quality community-based services for people with ID. As a senior lecturer, Sabah also contributed significantly to the teaching and the academic activities of the Section of UMDS at that time.

A most important development was that Geraldine Holt moved in 1990 from her post in Tower Hamlets to the Greenwich area of Oxleas Trust. She stayed there until 1996, when she moved to Lewisham and Guy's Mental Health NHS Trust to become a fully integrated member of the MHiLD team. Over the years, Geraldine Holt became a close colleague and a long-lasting family friend along with her husband Paul. She had started training in child psychiatry, which she interrupted to have a family, but she always wanted to specialise in ID. She was a graduate of the London Hospital Medical School and Sam Cohen, professor of psychiatry there, had requested that we develop a tailor-made training programme that would prepare Geraldine to be appointed as consultant psychiatrist in intellectual disabilities for the Tower Hamlets District in East London.

Geraldine's contribution to MHiLD was immense. She gave a new impetus to our services and had a marked influence on the important strategic and operational developments that followed. Geraldine took over the consultant psychiatrist responsibility of the MHiLD service for the Lewisham borough, while I remained responsible for Southwark. On a personal level, I had some relief from my intense service and academic commitments because for 15 years since my appointment I had been the single-handed consultant psychiatrist for North Southwark and Lewisham, in spite the fact that my contractual obligation was only for North Southwark! Geraldine was elected honorary secretary of the Faculty of LD of the Royal College of Psychiatrists from 2000 to 2004, and in 2005 she was seconded as senior policy advisor to the Department of Health. When Geraldine retired in July 2006 her valedictory event was a moving occasion for all of us at MHiLD with whom she had worked for so many years.

Shaun Gravestock was also trained in our higher specialist training scheme holding the post of lecturer and senior registrar. Shaun took up a consultant post in ID in Northumberland but he returned to become consultant psychiatrist at Greenwich (vacated by Geraldine Holt) in 1997, strengthening even more our extended network of specialists. With the retirement of Dr Rosalind Bates in the Bromley area, Dr Robert Winterhalder – who also was a product of our higher specialist training – took up the post. The presence of all of these consultant psychiatrist colleagues in the neighbouring areas was the outcome of the higher specialist training scheme in the psychiatry of ID that we had all contributed to develop together over the years. The contribution of other high-calibre multidisciplinary colleagues created an atmosphere of professional optimism in delivering a high-quality service to our population. The dedication and commitment of many professionals working for the

NHS in the UK has been a long-standing, unique and admirable aspect on all fronts.

In the meantime, MHiLD had been secured with the skilful support of Phil Woods, service manager, who steered carefully through the commissioning uncertainties as they popped up from time to time. Community-based therapeutic interventions had been refined and we were offering a wide range of clinical services, as well as being involved with a variety of teaching and training initiatives and applied as research projects. A major success was that Phil secured for us a new office base in the new modern Thomas Guy House, and the psychiatric services at Guy's, including the York Clinic, were transferred there. The input of Chris Laming, our administrator, and Mei Jones, the lead CPN, in organising this move was remarkable. In addition to Lewisham and North Southwark, the whole Southwark borough was added to our service, as well as Lambeth. We had already developed strong links with both newly added services, including in Lambeth, where since 1995 we had made another interim arrangement for consultant cover, as we did earlier for MIETS, when Lachlan Campbell had resigned from his post.

In 1998 MHiLD moved into modern offices of the ground floor of the new York Clinic at Thomas Guy House, where there were individual offices for consultant psychiatrists, trainees and junior doctors, CPNs and administrators. With the newly acquired premises, MHiLD had for the first time a critical mass of professionals working together from the same base. The inauguration of Thomas Guy House was made by the Queen on 18 March 1998, and MHiLD was represented at the opening ceremony by Geraldine Holt and Mei Jones. This was the second time I had been present at Guy's when the Queen visited, the first time being on 6 May 1976 for the celebration of the

Reflections on the Challenges of Psychiatry in the UK and Beyond

250th anniversary of Guy's and the inauguration of the Guy's Tower.

The strategy

The operational problems we faced with inpatient admissions continued to create a lot of pressure on our service, particularly as we were coming across new complex clinical issues with an increasing number of people falling into the area of mild or borderline ID and/or autistic spectrum disorders (ASD). In addition, as already mentioned, there were some people with ID and mental health needs or challenging behaviour who required extra support in their residential accommodation that was not available with the model of 'ordinary housing' that was developed.

There was a restructuring of the Lewisham and Guy's Mental Health Trust and the responsibility for managing the MHiLD service was given to the directorate of specialist services, together with the other specialist mental health services of CAMHS and addictions. Mark Allen, an experienced mental health manager, took over as director of services. Mark recognised the pressure on our services, and with the support of Peter Reading, the Trust's CEO, decided to start a new round of negotiations with Lambeth, Southwark and Lewisham Health Commissioning, where Doug Adams, the deputy director for mental health, was receptive to our plea for more support to MHiLD.

Then, I started discussions with Geraldine Holt and psychology colleagues Theresa Joyce and Barley Oliver and the idea was put forward of trying to work out a 'strategy' of service developments across our entire catchment area and to integrate clinical services, training and research. A few years earlier we had tried a similar idea with Jim Watson when, with the support of Lewisham Mencap, we applied to Guy's Hospital Special Trustees for funding, but we had not been successful. This time, we thought that if the idea of integrating clinical services, training and research/ development was accepted, we would encapsulate it in a framework of a 'virtual centre'. Mark Allen grasped the idea of developing such a strategy and he suggested that if funding was secured the centre would not be 'virtual' but 'real', and would be based at the renovated Munro Clinic at Guy's, where a development project to upgrade the clinic as a training and teaching centre for CAMHS was about to start.

We presented our strategy to Lambeth, Southwark and Lewisham Health Commissioning in early 1997. The main proposals were to further strengthen MHiLD, the development of a small inpatient unit, and provision of a number of 'specialist houses' in the local communities for people with ID and mental health needs and/or challenging behaviour. All of these services were to be integrated with training and research arms in the 'centre' framework, supported by the NHS (Lewisham and Guy's Mental Health Trust) and King's College London. This is an extract from the introduction of the 'Strategy':

'It is envisaged that the Centre will focus on the provision of good quality specialist community services to those service users who have additional mental health needs or additional needs in terms of challenging behaviour (where there is no diagnosable mental illness); and that this will be backed up by the provision of a small specialist assessment and treatment unit, practice-based programmes of teaching and training and relevant clinical research. The development of a Centre,

which brings together clinical skills, training and consultancy for staff and academic research into relevant issues, could provide the necessary focus for this.

Traditionally there has been something of a split between practice and research and this has not been helpful in moving services on. However, such initiatives need to be 'grounded' in service delivery if they are to continue to be effective in the longer term. A practice-based Centre is a logical development in the present circumstances, and one which could draw on the skills of current staff as well as draw in others. The three components of clinical skills, training and consultancy, and research / development can work together to produce a Centre to promote good-quality community services for this service user group. The Centre would provide clinical interventions and advice to services with regard to those service users with additional complex needs. This would take the form of assessment and treatment within a small, locally based specialist facility, within the generic adult mental health services; longer-term work with supported housing and hopefully the development of more houses designated for those with mental health / challenging behaviour needs and a continuation of the current clinical services to service users locally.

The lack of trained staff in local services gives this a high priority. Training needs to be carefully tailored to the staff receiving it, taking account of their individual service users and their own organisational issues. Training offered by the Centre would need to be on the basis of knowledge of the service users and their needs, the present skills and capacities of the staff team and the organisational structure in which they operate. It would also aim to work closely with those services that are supporting service users who have been enabled to return to a community service following a period of specialist assessment and treatment. The Centre will also offer academic degree programmes through the Academic Department of Psychiatry of the GKT Medical School. It can therefore offer comprehensive training for staff at all levels of service organisations. It can also include support to those trainees currently undergoing professional training (eg. clinical psychology, psychiatry and nursing) by providing access to an ongoing clinical academic program. This is seen as a crucial component, given the difficulties of recruiting qualified staff. Much of this training is currently being offered, but needs to become more focused and organised to increase effectiveness.

The Centre will have a strong research focus and will concentrate on those issues which have high priority as clinical service issues. This can include effectiveness of interventions, staffing and organisational issues as well as service evaluation. The focus on research will include evaluating new developments in clinical services. This form of infrastructure will provide the necessary support to ensure that the service can maintain its standards. The experience of the last decade and consideration of the current situation suggests that some action needs to be taken if services are not to 'drift' back to providing institutional services to those with the most complex needs. There needs to be a bringing together of the various strands, which are necessary to promote good quality community services to people with mental health needs and / or challenging behaviour.'

Following lengthy and intense but constructive negotiations over several months, Doug Adams of Lambeth, Southwark and Lewisham Health Commissioning (LSL) accepted the proposal for our strategy and was willing to identify ways of funding it. He needed, however, the agreement for the contribution of the other commissioners in the three boroughs, as their budgets would have to be 'top-sliced'. Doug organised a one-day seminar in the summer of 1997, and all stakeholders were invited to discuss the proposed strategy. The meeting was chaired by Glynis Murphy, at that time reader in applied psychology at the University of Kent, and, as mentioned in Chapter 5, a nationally and internationally renowned clinical psychologist in ID. Participants had been given copies of the strategy before the meeting and were invited to present their comments. After almost 20 years, it is interesting to look back at the comments made at that meeting. All supported the extension of the community function of MHiLD and the developments in training and research. However, the development of the inpatient unit and the 'specialist houses' was only supported by Southwark and Lambeth Social Services and Optimum HealthCare (representing occupational therapists and speech and language therapists); Lewisham Partnership was ambivalent and Lambeth Healthcare NHS Trust rejected the proposals. However, neither of the two organisations that did not support the strategy were able to offer any alternative proposal for how to solve the serious ongoing problems with admissions. This attitude, known as 'passing the parcel' or 'fudging the issues', was common in the NHS! Glynis Murphy was overall supportive of the strategy but mentioned that instead of having an inpatient unit we should consider 'developing a house' for admissions. I stated that this was not a viable solution.

The proposal of our strategy for the development of a Centre for Mental Health and ID was finally accepted in 1998 and the implementation started later the same year.[52] Jo Kent was assigned as the project manager. She and I had worked together previously on the Bexley Hospital re-provision of adult mental health services. Jo was a very experienced mental health manager and worked methodically and with enthusiasm to successfully implement the project. She was assisted by Mei Jones, our CPN lead, and together they used every available minute and made every effort to take through this important development. Mei had joined our service as a student nurse and after qualifying as a CPN returned to eventually become team leader. She was the driving force in creating a core group of CPN colleagues who contributed to the delivery of our service with immense skill and commitment.

Identifying space for the inpatient specialist unit became a problem that was eventually overcome by using a small ward of six beds that had remained unoccupied when the inpatient wards had moved from the York Clinic to Thomas Guy House. Though this space was not ideal for an inpatient specialist unit for people with ID, it was nevertheless an acceptable, realistic interim solution, until a better space could hopefully be found at a later stage. There was a great

---

52 The idea of developing an integrated centre of clinical services, training and research was adopted over 10 years later, with the creation of Clinical Academic Groups (CAGs) by King's Health Partners in London – a collaboration between King's College London, SLaM, and the Guy's, St Thomas' and King's College Hospital NHS Foundation Trusts.

deal of excitement about these new developments and this boosted the spirits of the MHiLD team, which now exceeded the minimum critical mass for a functioning unit and was composed of multidisciplinary mental health professionals specialising in meeting the needs of people with ID. The greatest benefit to service users, their families and carers was the provision of more comprehensive and locally based services.

The implementation of the strategy took over a year, with the community components and particularly the psychology and challenging needs specialists having been appointed first. Nurses for the inpatient unit followed, led by Mei Jones, as well as the appointment of Dr Kiriakos Xenitidis as half-time consultant for the new inpatient unit and half-time for MIETS. Jo Dwer led the input of occupational therapy. The staff roles were imaginative and flexible to allow most of them to work in the community and the inpatient unit. Following a lengthy discussion and search for an appropriate name, we settled eventually on the name of the street where the unit was located: the Weston Unit opened in June 1999. The aims of the Weston Unit was:

'... to provide a specialist assessment and treatment service within an appropriate environment for service users whose needs are not being met (this may be the result of a long length of stay on an acute ward, a residential placement which was breaking down, a private sector placement or over-provision in a forensic or challenging behaviour placement).'

Individualised packages of care were devised that combined multidisciplinary input from community services with intensive support from Weston Unit staff. Care plans included follow-up arrangements for people leaving the Weston Unit, in addition to the day-to-day plans relating to the stay on the unit. A coordinated approach was ensured between the Weston Unit, the community services and residential providers. Effective liaison was ensured with colleagues in adult mental health, adolescent services, forensic services, social services, housing departments, housing associations and voluntary agencies.

When the implementation of the strategy began, there were lengthy discussions and negotiations mostly with certain members of the psychology team about the numbers and the role of the nursing staff in the in-patient unit. These were successfully overcome by Jo Kent and Mei Jones, but led to much frustration and time-wasting. This is another example of individual agendas in the NHS being allowed to delay and distract from agreed and planned developments. The training and research developments of the strategy are presented in Chapter 10. The only part of the proposed strategy that was not implemented was the provision of 'specialist houses'. This was mainly because, following long discussions, the social services departments decided not to undertake the implementation of that part of the strategy – for reasons that never became clear but presumably had to do with funding. This was and remained a gap in the services, as there were a number of people with ID and complex mental health problems who after assessment and treatment required more intense and skilful support in their living environment.

While the strategy was in progress, Lewisham and Guy's Mental Health Trust and the Maudsley were merged together with Lambeth and Croydon Mental Health Services in 1998 to form the Foundation Trust of South London and Maudsley NHS (SLaM). Stuart Bell was appointed the new CEO and Mark Allen remained director of specialist services. Stuart Bell was leading what was then one of the largest mental health organisations in Europe, if not in the world, incorporating the prestigious Maudsley Hospital and the Institute of Psychiatry. The new SLaM Trust offered fresh momentum to all parts of local mental health services, including MHiLD; this momentum lasted for years and past my retirement.

The following year, 1999, was an *annus mirabilis* for me, as in addition to the new service developments, I was offered a personal chair as professor of psychiatry, following a two-year evaluation process that started with UMDS but was completed under King's College London. I was most grateful to Jim Watson for the nomination and to all the colleagues who supported me, including Peter Reading, CEO of the Lewisham and Guy's Mental Health Trust, and Dinshaw Master, then medical director.

Restructuring of the establishment of the services with the new SLaM Trust was unavoidable. There were now two services for the mental health problems of people with ID in the same trust: MHiLD and the MIETS Unit (see also Chapter 5). We had already developed strong links with colleagues at the MIETS Unit, in professional matters including the rotation of higher trainees, joint academic meetings and research, since Declan Murphy returned from the NIMH and was appointed consultant psychiatrist for MIETS.[53] Managerially and structurally, however, we belonged to different organisations. For a long time, I had been arguing that it would be beneficial to our field in South East London, and beyond, if MIETS and MHiLD joined in a single organisational structure. This idea resurfaced again with the creation of SLaM Trust, and discussions

---

53 Declan Murphy, professor of brain maturation at the Institute of Psychiatry and world-leading psychiatrist in neuroimaging for people with autistic spectrum disorders.

started about the best way to combine the expertise of MHiLD and MIETS.

With the implementation of the strategy and the expansion of our community mental health services, the Weston Unit and the Estia Centre (see Chapter 10) in full operation, we consolidated our position in SLaM as a specialist service for people with ID. The service had a critical mass of multidisciplinary mental health professionals with distinct skills and expertise. The addition of the Lambeth service, with David Brooks as consultant psychiatrist and the support and collaboration of Hedy Dicthfield, consultant psychologist, provided additional strength. However, we had once more to disentangle long historical issues of commissioning and budgets, this time in Lambeth.

The Weston Unit, led skillfully Mei Jones, provided assessment and treatment to those people with ID that needed admission. Though we did not cover every case requiring admission – having only six beds – we nevertheless covered a substantial part of the need and, in addition, we were able to transfer suitable people from the acute psychiatric wards. The Care Programme Approach (CPA) was fully implemented for all admissions to the Weston Unit and was gradually extended to community service users. It provided a systematic coordination and review of service users' care plans, which was for the most part accepted and appreciated by service users, families, carers, GPs in primary care, and social services.

The implementation of the CPA, however, created some difficulties with some of our psychologists, who expressed the view that people with ID falling in the blurred/overlapping area of challenging needs and psychiatric diagnosis should not to be included in the CPA process, even though they were receiving psychiatric input.

Consolidation of implementation

At the end of 2004 Mei Jones moved with her family to Wales. She left behind a noticeable gap, which was very successfully filled by Lynette Kennedy, CPN, who took over the team lead role. Lynette developed further the role of CPNs, and organised and steered the transfer of the Weston Unit to a more spacious environment at the Maudsley Hospital in 2004. From 2000 onwards, we had a coherent and established specialist service for people with ID and mental health needs. This was integrated with the robust training and research activities of the Estia Centre, which extended further locally, nationally and internationally. We were frequently invited to lecture and present our clinical experience, training initiatives and research findings at a variety of local, national and international events, including workshops, conferences and congresses (see also Chapter 10). Our work was greatly facilitated by the admirable and efficient support provided by Jenny Martin, senior administrator, who very successfully reorganised and improved the administrative systems and became a vital and integral part of MHiLD.

Soon after the turn of the new millennium, and while we were operationally going full steam ahead, a new joint commissioner in Southwark started again a pointless process to unilaterally commission MHiLD and separate the joined operation from the other boroughs, while transferring the management to social services. There was no justification whatsoever for this idea, which was alien to what had been built up over the years operating within SLaM, a major mental health NHS Foundation Trust in collaboration with King's College London. Because of this issue, we wasted precious time with Mark Allen, the director of our services, in discussions and negotiations for over two years until the individual in question moved on to another job in another part of the country and the problem was consequentially resolved. Over the years, I found it incomprehensible, as I have already stated, that such issues were allowed to create entirely unnecessary problems and obstacles in the NHS, and waste costly time and resources.

In the following years, there were some important changes to the membership of the staff group.[54] They took part in a wide range of teaching, training and research activities, which were service-oriented and aimed to improve the quality of local services on an evidence base.

In 2005 we were invited to tender – and put in a successful bid – for the mental health service for people with ID for the Croydon borough, whose generic mental health services were already provided by SLaM. Furthermore, the newly appointed consultant psychiatrists for Croydon were already working closely with us. This contract started in April 2006 and extended the MHiLD services across the four boroughs of Lambeth, Southwark, Lewisham and Croydon. A new series of discussions and negotiations started again, with local commissioners looking at another chain of historical commissions, arrangements and agreements among different parts of services.

The MHiLD service was innovative in its concept as a focus on specialist mental health provision for

---

54 David Brooks left in 2004 to take up a consultant post in Lincoln and was succeeded by Jean O'Hara, who moved to our service from Tower Hamlets. Max Pickard, having completed his training with us, was appointed as consultant psychiatrist in Croydon in 2003 and Jane McCarthy was appointed as a second consultant psychiatrist in Croydon in 2004. Colin Hemmings was appointed in 2004 as consultant psychiatrist for Lewisham, as Geraldine Holt was seconded to the Department of Health as Policy Advisor. The new colleagues, together with Andrew Flynn, consultant psychiatrist in Bexley, became important members of the Estia Centre.

local people with ID within a generic mental health organisation, integrated with a training arm and a clinically oriented research/development arm. The MHiLD model had at its core a person-centred approach and a value base that promoted social inclusion and independence, as well as integration with generic services. There were examples of good cross-working with adult mental health services, both in inpatient and community settings for people with ID and acute mental health problems accessing the same range of local provision as everyone else, with specialist support and facilitation as required. At the same time, MHiLD provided specialist supports for those whose complex presentation meant that using generic mental health services was neither possible nor desirable. Multidisciplinary community-based interventions were the predominant mode of operation, with the CPNs at the core of the team. Outpatient clinics were running in various outpatient departments, and those in need of inpatient care were admitted to the Weston Unit for assessment and treatment. Therapeutic interventions included medication and environmental manipulation, as well as psychological treatments such as anxiety management and cognitive-behavioural therapy.

At the same time, MHiLD had been accepted as one of the specialist services of SLaM, as a cohesive team that was fully compliant with clinical governance requirements. We held weekly clinical meetings; implemented the Care Programme Approach (CPA) with as much service users participation as possible; carried out regular audit meetings, which were presented at trust-wide events; and supported the personal development of all members of staff. The CPA framework was particularly useful, as it provided a single care plan that considered risk assessment and management, including crisis and contingency plans and future reviews. MHiLD had developed a combination of secondary and tertiary care functions for the mental health needs of people with ID, as well as strong interfaces with generic mental health services. This type of model not only provided a specialist service, but was designed to complement existing services through its interfaces with both generic adult mental health and community ID services. It provided information on appropriate assessment and treatment strategies, but also offered practical assistance to acute and other general mental health services.

Further developments

In spite of the implementation of the strategy described above, and the progress in the delivery of services, two issues continued to require serious attention, particularly in view of the ever changing service demands. These were:

a. The organisation and structure related to the reconfiguration of MHiLD, with the MIETS Unit and the Behavioural Disorders Unit (BDU) all being part of SLaM.

b. The interface between MHiLD and forensic adult mental health services. The BDU was an inpatient unit, based at Bethlem Royal Hospital, for people with challenging behaviour but without ID.

There was intense concern about these issues from 2002 to 2007. This was prompted following my annual appraisal by David Roy, then SLaM medical director, and Tom Craig, professor of community and social psychiatry. Having dual clinical and academic responsibilities, my annual appraisal was conducted jointly by senior colleagues from the NHS and the medical school. They both thought that there were serious service issues that needed top-level management attention. Twice in recent months Stuart Bell, SLaM CEO, had been subpoenaed to court because two people with mild ID needed admission to a forensic unit and none of the existing services were able to accept them. In a constructive meeting initiated by David Roy and attended by Stuart Bell, Mark Allen and I, the decision was made to set up two working groups with senior members of the trust, to make recommendations for the reconfiguration of the services and the interface with adult forensic mental health. For that purpose, Eddie Chaplin, an experienced nurse manager, who became an integral member of MHiLD and the Estia Centre, was seconded from the MIETS Unit to MHiLD in late 2004, and Sue Culling was appointed as operational manager in 2005. Sue was a very methodical and organised manager who understood problems quickly and tried to facilitate workable solutions. In addition, Peter Gluckman, one of the local NHS 'grandees', was brought in from the local primary care trust to chair the working group on forensic ID. Louise Adams, SLaM's senior developments manager, served the working group. It was a top-level management activity. At that time SLaM had a trust-wide Forensic Strategy Group chaired by Stuart Bell, with Ann Watts as project manager and Andrew Johns, consultant forensic psychiatrist, planning major developments in forensic services, including a medium secure unit at the Bethlem Hospital. The ID Forensic and Complex Development Project Group became a subgroup of the SLaM Forensic Strategy Group. This was a time of intense work but also of high optimism that difficult issues related to mental health care of people with ID, including those with complex forensic needs, was being addressed at such a high management level. This allowed us to have hope that workable solutions would emerge.

The specialist mental health Weston Unit (six beds for the whole of Lambeth, Southwark and Lewisham) for people with mild/moderate intellectual disabilities and mental health needs had reduced the necessity of sending people out of borough to specialist units for assessment and treatment. It had also provided a significant relief for admissions to generic adult mental health wards. Furthermore, it had developed expertise to assess and offer treatment/care plans to service users with ID and very complex mental health needs, such as autistic spectrum disorders and additional psychiatric disorders. However, the Weston Unit had neither absorbed all admissions to generic adult mental health wards, nor cared for people with ID and forensic and complex needs.[55] At that time a publication from the voluntary organisation the Judith Trust[56] recommended 12 specialist admission and treatment beds for the size of our catchment area.

The reconfiguration

It was necessary to try and build up a care pathway to meet local needs and stop out of area placements. This needed to be a mix of hospital-based and residential services. The needs of the three boroughs – Lambeth, Lewisham and Southwark – were different. The findings, based on an internal review of available clinical data over a two-to-five-year projection, anticipated that overall, in all three boroughs, there would be a decrease in the need for medium secure

---

55 Bouras N, Holt G, Murphy D, Brooks D, Xenitidis K (2001) Mental health services for people with learning disabilities. *Psychiatric Bulletin* **25** 323.

56 http://www.judithtrust.org.uk/

unit ID services, whereas the need for residential services for the ID forensic and complex group would increase. These predictions demonstrated the need for a range of provision, which was challenging, given the relatively small numbers. Also not to be forgotten were new entries, which again further illustrated demand for specialist services. The outline recommendations included reconfiguration of the MIETS Unit and of the Weston Unit into a single management structure. MIETS would become the main inpatient admission unit while the Weston Unit would have a step-down function for service users admitted to MIETS, and would also remain as a specialist assessment and treatment unit. A range of enhanced and highly structured residential facilities would be required, as well as strengthening of the existing community-based specialist services to support service users in residential facilities, providing in-reach into generic services to facilitate discharge from inpatient units, preventing new admissions, and delivering skills-based and awareness training.

The merger of MHiLD and MIETS was never implemented and operational autonomy was maintained with two clinical directors! One of the main reasons for not merging the two services was that MIETS had a commissioning system that differed from the commissioning of local services. The MIETS commissioning was partially from the national specialist services and partially from extra-contractual referrals (known as ECRs). In addition to MIETS, SLaM had another inpatient unit, the BDU at Bethlem Royal Hospital, for people with challenging behaviour without ID. These two inpatient units shared certain service similarities and were under one management structure. An important recommendation at that time was for the MHiLD service to work together with the Weston Unit,

MIETS and BDU. They were to extend their provision to people with autistic spectrum disorders and become a 'neurodevelopmental disorders service'. The concept of converting the mental health services for those with ID to a service for neurodevelopmental disorders was thought to be relevant because of the increasing number of people referred to our service with autistic spectrum disorder, including Asperger's. A specialist mental health service like MHiLD was considered to be more able to meet these people's needs than a generic mental health service.

Though the proposed idea was received with interest from the management of SLaM and was discussed in detail, and also received support from social services and some commissioners, it was never implemented. It is clear from the description of the recommended services that the development of admission facilities was always only one part of the proposals, and that there was always more emphasis on the development of appropriate supported accommodation and related enhanced community supports.

Interface and forensic

The interface with adult forensic mental health services addressed examined the following groups of service users:

- First, some people who had attended special schools also had severe psychiatric illness and were under adult mental health services; they functioned at borderline cognitive impairment level but presented with some difficult diagnostic and treatment problems requiring MHiLD input.

- Second, people who had attended special schools

and had been functioning at the borderline cognitive impairment level and presented with poor impulse control, and might or might not have had a personality disorder, could end up in the forensic adult mental health service and require specialist MHiLD input, because of difficult diagnostic and treatment problems.

■ Third, an increasing number of people with autistic spectrum disorders, including Asperger's syndrome, who might have fulfilled the eligibility criteria for ID services or have been functioning at the borderline cognitive impairment level, and were under the remit of adult mental health services.

■ Fourth, those people with ID and complex mental health needs who were placed 'historically' out of area, mostly by the different social services departments in private 'assessment and treatment' facilities at major expense for all concerned.

Furthermore, the failure to develop specialist supported housing – the provision of which had been part of our strategy – continued, perpetuating the problem of moving service users out of area to expensive private facilities, often for several years, for residential care. This continues to be a major problem, even in 2017. It was estimated at that time that £8.8 million was spent from local services on this service users' group for out of area placements. Approximately £4.3 million (49% of the total) was spent by social services and £4.5 million (51%) by SLaM, although health and social services figures, as a proportion, varied across boroughs.

The ID Forensic and Complex Development Project group worked intensively for six months in 2005/6. The group's recommendations included:

■ forming a joint management forum (AMH/ID Forum) in each borough to manage resources associated with the existing and new ID forensic entries

■ protocols and eligibility criteria between services

■ the need for a reinvestment pool of the then current expenditure

■ to create a focal point for information and recommendations regarding clinical information and implications of the forensic and complex project

■ to take a strategic view of current situations and future need, and developments for forensic and complex ID service users

■ assessment of all forensic and complex ID service users who were out of area

■ to conduct a range of predetermined assessments to inform future placement advice and management strategies

■ to assume a staff development role for nurses undertaking assessment and discharge work

■ to assist in standard-setting and evaluating quality outcomes

■ to access the capacity of existing services

■ to provide a framework for involving all parties in the context of long-term strategic planning and investment, while acknowledging and tackling the barriers that exist to truly effective joint working.

In March 2007 a one-day seminar was organised by SLaM. It was chaired by Stuart Bell, CEO of SLaM, and attended by senior managers and clinicians. The aim was to discuss the recommendations and the implementation of the trust-wide forensic strategy. By the time of my retirement, the new medium secure unit at Bethlem Hospital had been commissioned for the adult forensic mental health services but no provision was made in the new unit for people with ID. The related issues were once more left unresolved and on the shelf! The efforts to reconfigure the inpatient units of the Weston Unit, MIETS and BDU met the same fate, and they remained functioning separately. This is another example of the paradoxes seen in the NHS that are difficult to understand on face validity. I think that what is even more difficult, is to identify the lines of accountability. Several reconfigurations of these services took place at later stages after my retirement –but these are not the subject of this book.[57] The review of the Care Quality Commission (CQC) at the time of writing rated the MHiLD service as outstanding.

Meeting the mental health needs of people with ID remains a challenge for everyone. There has been an increasing tendency to access mainstream community and inpatient assessment, treatment, forensic and rehabilitation facilities with a varied level of success. This trend needs to continue and to be strengthened, but a degree of specialisation will be necessary. The provision of special mental health services will depend on local developments and services. Strong inter-agency communication among the health, social and voluntary sectors will also be crucial, as well as providing support services to meet residential, recreational and vocational needs. Service user and carer participation is of utmost importance, in order to ensure that suitable and appropriate priorities are set and that services are satisfactorily provided.

---

57 After my retirement MIETS and the Weston Unit integrated into a single unit. This resulting unit came together with BDU under one structure and was streamlined into a 'Neurodevelopmental Disorders Pathway' with one clinical director.

Chapter 10:
The Estia Centre

The Estia Centre was established at the end of 1999 as part of the strategy (see also Chapter 9) and presented an innovative development in the field of ID. We initially appointed a research coordinator, a training coordinator, a development manager and an administrator. The third floor of the newly refurbished Munro Clinic at Guy's (renamed the Munro Centre) became the base of the Estia Centre, as it had several offices and on-site access to lecture rooms equipped with IT technology that was state of the art at the time. Steve Hardy was appointed as training coordinator and soon became the key person overseeing the training initiatives of the Estia Centre. Steve later undertook the management of the centre and very successfully organised and delivered a wide range of training and educational programmes that contributed to the national and international recognition of the Estia Centre. The centre held a launch on 27 January 2000, and this was attended by senior colleagues of SLaM and the Institute of Psychiatry (IoP), including the CEO Stuart Bell and Professor Graham Thornicroft, chairman of the Health Service and Population Research Department of the IoP. Both praised the development of the Estia Centre and pledged their support. Speakers at the launch included Steve Moss on 'The relationship of challenging

behaviour to psychiatric symptomatology', Declan
Murphy on 'Brain studies and challenging behaviour',
Glynis Murphy on 'Issues of risk and consent' and
Theresa Joyce on 'Outcomes and challenging behaviour
in community services. Together with Geraldine
Holt and Hedy Ditchfield, I outlined the importance
of specialist mental health services for people with
ID and acknowledged the decisive contribution of
Mark Allen, director of services, and Jo Kent, project
manager, in the realisation of the Estia Centre.

The Estia Centre grew to be the hub and focus of
all our training, teaching and research/development
activities, and these were fully integrated with the
clinical services. We transferred functionally to the
Estia Centre all the activities that we had previously
operated from the Section of Mental Health in Learning
Disabilities, and we expanded our portfolio of research
and development. We gradually shaped the structure of
the Estia Centre to have three work streams: training,
led by Geraldine Holt, which was divided into training
and dissemination, MSc and postgraduate diploma,
and consultancy; service user involvement, led initially
by Ann Faulkner and then Steve Hardy and Eddie
Chaplin; and research and development, led by Helen
Costello and myself.

Teaching and learning

The MSc in Mental Health of Learning Disabilities
(MSc-MHLD) evolved over the years from an optional
module of the MSc in mental health studies offered
by the Division of Psychiatry and Psychology of the
UMDS in 1996, to an approved separate taught course
obtainable from the IoP of King's College London
in 2005 (See also Chapter 11). The MSc-MHLD was
well subscribed and became a significant source of

income, which subsidised the research projects of the Estia Centre. Several colleagues had a key role in organising and delivering the MSc-MHLD, including Paula McAlpine, Steve Higgins, Rob Winterhalder, Steve Hardy, Elias Tsakanikos and Eddie Chaplin. Elias Tsakanikos was appointed as lecturer in 2005, and reorganised the curriculum and raised the academic standards of the course.

The MSc-MHLD was designed to provide continuing professional development for mental health and ID professionals, as well as up-to-date knowledge and understanding of mental health issues for psychology graduates with academic and/or clinical interests in the area of ID. The MSc-MHLD consisted of five modules: basic mental health, research methods, two specialist ID modules and a dissertation. The specialist modules covered aetiology, psychopathology and assessment, the theoretical and empirical basis of clinical management of mental health needs, forensic issues and services, neurodevelopmental aspects; and pervasive developmental disorders. The programme was delivered by a wide range of visiting lecturers – academic and clinical experts in mental health and ID. There were established links with active research groups at the IoP so that students could undertake their MSc dissertation under the supervision of experienced clinical or academic researchers.

Training initiatives

The Estia Centre was commissioned to offer training to organisations that provided care and support to people with ID and additional mental health needs and/or challenging needs (renamed from challenging behaviour) across the London boroughs of Lambeth, Lewisham and Southwark. It also provided training to external agencies, either independently or in collaboration with other providers. The training courses were developed and delivered by staff from the Estia Centre in close collaboration with clinical staff. The main aim was to support family carers, support staff and health and social care professionals to be competent in promoting positive mental health, identifying mental health problems, and accessing and providing appropriate services and interventions for people with ID. Until the introduction of the formal vocational qualifications specific to people with ID in 2001, support staff often had no formal qualifications in health or social care. This was a significant mismatch, given their role in providing some of the most important aspects for maintaining a person's quality of life. In developing the Estia Centre training programme, we initially completed a training needs analysis with local service providers. We also consulted local groups of people with ID, and professionals from the local community and CMHTs. This resulted in a rolling programme of workshops that were provided free of charge to local not-for-profit services.

Workshops were developed with input from a range of disciplines and from people using services. The content reflected the evidence base of the subject and current policy. Workshops were based around a framework of skills and knowledge that participants should possess in order to provide effective care in different care settings. These included support staff working in social care housing with individuals who had identified mental health problems and healthcare assistants, as well as support staff working in specialist assessment and treatment services.

The Estia Centre offered workshops on mental health and associated issues, such as activities and skills development, the Mental Capacity Act, introduction to autism, introduction to challenging needs, mental health for adults with ID, mental health and older people with ID, risk around an individual, risk assessment and management for senior staff, self-injurious behaviour, and using objects, photos and symbols as aids to communication and independence for people with ID.

The training package

Many of the materials used in the training programmes were based on the Estia Centre publication *Mental Health in Learning Disabilities: A training resource*.[58] This is a comprehensive programme, consisting of over 70 hours of learning activities, which are split into 18 themed modules. It provides trainers with detailed lecture notes, slides, handouts, various learning activities and video case vignettes. Trainers are also provided with an accompanying reader which gives detailed supporting information for each module. The training pack *Mental Health in Learning Disabilities* was first published in 1995 as part of our training activities and before having formally established the Estia Centre. The training pack reached three editions.[59] In 1993 we received a small grant towards the publication from the Department of Health and it took us two years to develop the material. The pack represented an innovative training concept and it became hugely successful. Pavilion Publishing, led at that time by Jan Alcoe and Chris Parker, published the training package and continued doing so in its

58 Holt G, Hardy S & Bouras N (2005) *Mental Health in Learning Disabilities: A training resource*. Brighton: Pavilion Publishing.

59 Bouras N, Murray B & Joyce T (eds) (1995) *Mental Health in Learning Disabilities Training Package*. Brighton: Pavilion Publishing.

subsequent editions. The launch of the first edition took place at the NADD International Congress in Boston in 1995. It attracted much interest, which stimulated an edition adapted to US requirements.[60] There was also an edition adapted for Australian requirements,[61] and the training pack was also translated into Greek.

The Estia Centre has produced several other publications in the form of practical guides for support and related staff. Many of these were produced in collaboration with other organisations. For example, *Supporting Complex Needs* was produced in collaboration with the charity Turning Point. It offered a proactive approach to meeting mental health needs, empowering support staff to recognise their own valued role in implementing high-quality support for service users with ID.[62] Other practical publications of the Estia Centre included a self-help guide that enabled staff to develop strategies for supporting those with challenging behaviour, by offering realistic information and guidance on how to work with other professionals.[63] Both people who used services and support staff were involved in the development of these publications.

Another initiative by the Estia Centre was the publication of a comprehensive guide on mental health

60 Cain N, Holt G, Davidson P & Bouras N (2006) *Training Handbook of Mental Disorders in Individuals with Intellectual Disability*. New York: NADD Press.

61 Edwards N, Lennox N, Holt G & Bouras N (2003) *Mental Health in Adult Developmental Disability: Education and training kit for professionals and service providers*. Brisbane: QICIDD, University of Queensland.

62 Hardy S, Kramer R, Holt G, Woodward P & Chaplin E (2006) *Supporting Complex Needs: A practical guide for support staff working with people with a learning disability who have mental health needs*. London: Turning Point.

63 Woodward P, Hardy S & Joyce T (2007) *Keeping it Together: A guide for support staff working with people whose behaviour is challenging*. Brighton: Pavilion Publishing and Media.

for families and carers of people with ID.[64] This guide was developed in consultation with family carers and people with ID, and focused on what people wanted to know regarding their family members' mental health, how to recognise possible mental health problems, how and when to access services, the range of available treatments, and how carers can help themselves. Case vignettes were used to illustrate both how mental health problems can affect the individual with ID, and the difficulties and dilemmas that carers face. The guide was evaluated by residential and day service providers, carers and service users. A quasi-experimental study demonstrated the role of training materials in increasing carer awareness of mental health problems and improving the psychiatric outcome of individuals with ID. The guide was highly commended in 2004 by the National Institute for Mental Health in England (NIMHE) in the category of Positive Practice Awards.

The Estia Centre also published evaluation studies that proved the effectiveness of its methods used in training support staff.[65] A comprehensive review of the training activities of the Estia Centre was written by Helen Costello and colleagues and included in a special publication to mark my retirement.[66]

64 Holt G, Gratsa A, Bouras N, Joyce T, Spiller MJ & Hardy S (2004) *Guide to Mental Health for Families and Carers of People with Intellectual Disabilities.* London: Jessica Kingsley.

65 Costello H, Bouras N & Davis H (2007) The role of training in improving community care staff awareness of mental health problems in people with intellectual disabilities. *Journal of Applied Research in Intellectual Disabilities* **20** 228–235.

66 Costello H, Hardy S, Tsakanikos E & McCarthy J (2010) Training professionals, family carers and support staff to work effectively with people with intellectual disability and mental health problems. In: N Bouras and G Holt (eds) *Mental Health Services for Adults with Intellectual Disability: Strategies and solutions.* Hove: Psychology Press.

External seminars and workshops

Long before the Estia Centre had been set up, the interest that MHiLD and training initiatives attracted had motivated us to organise educational and training events for professionals and support staff at regional, national and international levels.

The first of such events was a one-day conference organised at Guy's in 1988, entitled 'Current Themes in Mental Health and Mental Handicap'. This included presentations and workshops, mostly on practical topics and delivered by our members of staff but also by invited experts with a national reputation. Current Themes in Mental Health and Mental Handicap became a regular annual event (always with a full house) held at the Robens Suite in the Guy's Tower, which has a spectacular view of the Tower Bridge and the Thames.

In 1993 we were invited by the Institute of Public Health South East Thames to participate in a series of conferences and seminars. These were initially held locally but were soon extended nationally. The events were very successful and included topics such as 'Learning disabilities: measuring outcomes-quality assurance', 'LD, sexuality and society', 'Residential and day services', 'Future provision of services', 'Employment opportunities and daytime activities', 'Older people with LD', 'Stress and staff', 'The criminal justice system', etc. A special publication on commissioning and providing mental health services for people with ID was also published jointly with the Institute of Public Health.[67]

In 1998 the Institute of Public Health ceased its educational activities and the organisation of the conferences and seminars was taken over by Conference

---

67 Bouras N & Dolan P (1997) *Challenges and Change: Commissioning and providing services for people with learning disabilities.*

Administration and Training Services (CATS), led by Nicola Murray, who had previously run these events for the Institute of Public Health. We delivered several conferences; one of the most interesting was held at the Royal Society of Medicine in celebration of the 50th anniversary of the NHS. It was themed around 'Achievements, Difficulties, and the Future of Services for People with Learning Disabilities'. The conference was attended by many colleagues, clinicians and managers. It is worth noting that in my talk I pointed out that institutions for people with ID would soon belong to the past. A senior clinical colleague criticised me, saying that my presentation was provocative when I stated that the long-stay institutions were about to close! CATS stopped working in 1999 when we set up the Estia Centre and all of these activities were relocated there.

Following the publication of the training package, in 1997 we started collaborating with Pavilion Publishing on a series of successful multidisciplinary educational programmes and a number of national conferences and seminars. These events were initially held at the ORT Centre in North London or the Robens Suite at Guy's. They were organised either independently, jointly with Pavilion, or in collaboration with other organisations in London or other parts of the UK and Ireland. With the development of the Estia Centre, these activities became part of the training and education portfolio of the centre. The programme included 'Team-centred Training', which was delivered to a particular staff team and specifically tailored for their service's needs; 'Service User-centred Training', on the needs of a particular service user and delivered with the involvement of a clinician known to the service user; and training that covered several other topics, including 'Understanding the Mental Health Act (1983)' and its 'Implications for Service Users, Carers and Staff; and Working with Offenders who have LD'.

The Estia Centre's collaboration with Pavilion Publishing continued, delivering an extensive programme of national conferences and seminars, sometimes jointly with other organisations, on the mental health needs of people with learning disabilities and associated issues, for example; 'Listening More Carefully to the Needs of People with Both Mental Health Problems and LD', in collaboration with the National Development Team, in 2000; 'Autism: A review of current controversies in LD', and 'Clinical and Social Challenges of Aggressive Behaviour in LD', in 2001. National seminars were also held in collaboration with Professor Peter Sturmey, an associate collaborator of the Estia Centre from City University of New York, and Matt Janicki of IASSIDD. Topics of some other national conferences organised by the Estia Centre included 'Challenging Behaviour: Refocusing', which examined best practice in meeting the challenging needs of people with LD (held in 2001); 'Practice Consensus in Dual Diagnosis: Anxiety disorders', which examined the evidence base and best practice in working with people with LD who had anxiety disorders (2002); 'Meeting the Mental Health Needs of Women with LD', a national seminar held in collaboration with the Judith Trust (2002); 'Mental Health and People with LD: Clinical directions from *Valuing People*' (2003); 'Forensic Learning Disabilities: Specialist services for people with complex needs' (2004); 'Meeting the Mental Health Needs of People with Learning Disabilities: Approaches to diversity' (2004). In 2001 the Estia Centre published the *Mini-PAS-ADD* assessment tool, in collaboration with Pavilion Publishing. It was very well received. All of the training and educational activities described above were evidence-based practice. The aim of these activities was to develop the skills of multidisciplinary staff members to enable them to effectively support service users with a wide range of mental health needs.

The Estia Centre also undertook the organisation of a monthly multidisciplinary programme at Guy's. This was free of charge and open to any local and regional professionals supporting people with ID. The programme consisted of a case presentation, a publications review, a research project review and a lecture by an invited speaker. Topics varied in nature but aimed to keep staff up-to-date with recent developments in policy and practice. This programme became very successful locally and regionally, and we had to ask people to register to avoid overcrowding. The invited speakers include many well-known experts in ID.[68]

Advances in mental health in learning disabilities

In 2007 the Estia Centre launched with Pavilion Publishing a new journal entitled *Advances in Mental Health in Learning Disabilities*. The aim was for the journal to be a high-quality resource on the mental health needs of people with ID, for practitioners, managers and academics. The idea was to integrate current research with practice, and keep professionals up-to-date with a variety of different perspectives on developments in the field. The journal aimed to support professionals in delivering high-quality and evidence-based practice to people with intellectual disabilities with additional mental health needs, and to provide a forum for debate on current issues and opinions.

---

68 For example; Professor Richard Hastings of Bangor University, Linda Jordan of the Valuing People Support Team, Hazel Morgan and Barbara McIntosh of the Foundation for People with Learning Disabilities, Professor Angela Hassiotis of University College London, Andrew Lee of People First, and many others who presented on their areas of expertise.

The contents of the journal included policy and its implications for practice, developments in service design and delivery, brief research reports and related service initiatives, clinical case studies that would enable professionals to learn from the experience of others and improve their own practice, opinions and debates, and book reviews. The first editors were Geraldine Holt and Steve Hardy, while I held the position of editorial advisor, supported by an international editorial advisory board. The journal became very successful thanks to the invaluable contribution of Steve Hardy, and continues to be published today with new editors and now renamed *Advances in Mental Health and Intellectual Disabilities*.

Research and development

The research and development (R&D) programme of the Estia Centre was service-orientated, and incorporated service evaluation, studies of the effectiveness of training and projects measuring clinical outcomes. These included studies of clinical effectiveness, staffing and organisational issues, the detection and diagnosis of mental health problems, and the use of psychological treatments. The research questions were defined on the basis of current clinical practice, and the need to address specific issues to ensure implementation of comprehensive clinical/support care packages. Research was conducted on local, regional, national and international bases.

One important step of setting up a new facility is to regularly collect information on the kind of provisions provided and the characteristics and needs of those who will use the service. At the start of our specialist community mental health service we adopted the same method used at the MHAC (see Chapter 2) of systematically monitoring all new referrals on a specially devised form, the Mental Health Assessment and Information Rating Profile that had been adapted from the first used Multi-axial and Information Rating Profile (see also Chapter 5).[69] This was before the digital era and the introduction of electronic medical records for the collection of routine clinical and service data. There was at that time a gross lack of information systems. Only Lewisham Social Services had a 'register', but that was out of date.

With the information recorded in the Mental Health Assessment and Information Rating Profile, service research studies were carried out over the years including all new referrals to our clinical service. The studies focused on emerging trends in referrals and pathways to care, the characteristics of service users referred to the specialist service and their consumption of services, as well as many others. These studies provided an important basis for an informed examination of the crucial question of whether there should be specialist or generic provision for people with mental health needs and ID. Studies looked at inpatient and community care, particularly for those with ID and additional severe psychiatric illness who at times needed more intensive support to be maintained in the community. Early publications were focused on a description of our six years' experience of running our community-based specialist mental health service for people with ID, and these attracted a lot of interest. We were flooded by requests for reprints from all over the world, as there was a paucity of similar studies at that time.[70] The then leading professor of psychiatry of ID, Joan Bicknell, wrote about this publication:

---

69 Bouras N & Drummond K (1989) Community psychiatric services in mental handicap. *Health Trends* **21** 72–78.

70 Bouras N, Drummond C, Brooks D & Laws M (1988) *Mental Handicap and Mental Health: A community service*. London: NUPRD.

*'It is probably the first of its kind to be made
available to a wide audience and attempt is made
to provide objective data on symptomatology of
people with mental handicap and mental illness
… if more teams (including my own) were to set
time aside for such an honest appraisal of the early
years of a team, knowledge of the psychiatric needs
of those people with a mental handicap who have
always lived in the community and those who are
coming out of the institutions to join them, would be
a lot more substantial.'* [71]

Several studies were published in peer review journals,
working papers and short publications. These were
based on a wide range of health service research
areas, such as the characteristics of service users and
consumption of services, referral pathways to care of
people with ID as well as autistic spectrum disorders,
exploration of ethnic factors in those referred to the
specialist mental health service, behaviour management
problems as predictors of using psychotropic medication,
use of psychiatric consultation and inpatient admission,
predictive factors for psychiatric inpatient admissions,
evaluation of the effectiveness of a specialist ID mental
health inpatient unit, and several others.

The Estia Centre conducted a number of
retrospective analyses that focused on the prevalence
of mental health problems, the vulnerabilities of
specific groups for developing mental health problems
and the characteristics of service provision. These
included studies examining risk factors for developing
psychopathology, risk factors for inpatient admission,
the relationship between mental health problems
and challenging behaviour, a comparison of psychotic

---

71 Bicknell J (1989) Mental handicap and community services.
Psychiatric Bulletin **13** (5) 267.

disorders in people with and without intellectual disabilities, psychopathology in individuals with pervasive developmental disorders, the role of life events in predicting psychopathology, referral trends, and risk factors for high mental health service utilisation.

Evidence about the effectiveness of generic and specialist mental health services for people with ID was sparse. To address this lack in the evidence base, the Estia Centre conducted a prospective study comparing the characteristics of individuals with ID who were admitted to generic inpatient services, compared to those admitted to specialist services.[72] The study found that individuals with ID who were admitted to a specialist unit demonstrated significant improvements in functioning, behaviours and psychopathology. The specialist unit was associated with significantly longer periods of admission, although discharge to expensive, out-of-area residential placements was less likely. Parallel qualitative studies were also conducted, which examined the interface between generic and specialist inpatient services, and explored the attitudes of staff within generic services in relation to meeting the mental health needs of people with ID. Estia Centre research also examined service user and carer perspectives and their levels of satisfaction with services.[73]

---

72 Xenitidis K, Gratsa A, Bouras N, Hammond R, Ditchfield H, Holt G, Martin J & Brooks D (2004) Psychiatric inpatient care for adults with intellectual disabilities: generic or specialist units? *Journal Intellectual Disability Research* **48** (1) 11–8.

73 I would like to acknowledge the commitment of colleagues over the years for their contribution to broadening the evidence base. Particularly notable are the contributions of Helen Costello and Elias Tsakanikos, who devised most of the research projects at the Estia Centre and made the best use of the collected information through their analysis. Important contributions, which have been documented in a series of publications, were also made by the research assistants Graham Martin, Lisa Underwood, Mary Spiller, Anastasia Gratsa, Amy Cowley, Charlie Maitland Fay Coster, Stephen Wright and others.

R&D at the Estia Centre was strengthened with the collaboration of external colleagues and departments. One of the most important links we developed was with Steve Moss, the creator of *PAS-ADD*, which remains to this day the most advanced diagnostic assessment method for mental health problems for people with ID. Steve joined the Section of LD at UMDS as an associate member in 1997, following the closure of the Hester Adrian Research Centre in Manchester. He gave a new impetus to our research work and contributed to the development of the research strategy of the Estia Centre when it started in 1999. Steve was part of a successful European Union grant that the centre obtained in 1998, as part of the BIOMED II programme on 'Improving the Detection of Mental Health Problems in People with Mental Retardation'. We named this project MEROPE, after a star in the Perseides who, according to Greek mythology, shone dimly because she had married Sisyphus, a mortal man. MEROPE was used as a metaphor for disability, that is, a star with a low shine but which is among others (integration). This was an exciting time for our research team, and we were collaborating with other partners in the project: Luis Salvador-Carulla from Spain, John Tsiantis from Greece, John Hillery from Ireland and Germain Weber from Austria. Many gaps were identified in relation to the generic mental health service provision in these countries, which was frequently found to be ad hoc and dependent on the goodwill and personal commitment of the professionals and volunteers involved. Service planning and policy formulation was found to be hindered by a lack of standardised diagnostic criteria, and effective interventions and policy and legislation had tended to separate the disability aspects of people with

ID from their mental health needs.[74]

Unfortunately, two other very carefully prepared applications led by Steve Moss and submitted to the European Union programmes were not successful – and the feedback we received was entirely irrelevant to the aims of the proposed research. At that time, research proposals to European Union programmes for people with ID were assessed by an expert group on 'disability', which dealt with all kinds of disabilities but mostly physical ones; a research proposal on the assessment of mental health problems for people with ID was alien to this expert group. The collaboration of Steve Moss with the Estia Centre continued for several years, even after my retirement, with Steve delivering training in the use of the *Mini PAS-ADD*. There was also close collaboration with Steve Moss on other international projects and organisations that are mentioned in Chapter 12.

The Estia Centre either led or participated as a collaborator in several research projects funded by national and international bodies. A very significant source of R&D funding was the Special Trustees of Guy's and St Thomas' hospitals, or Guy's and St Thomas' Charity, as it is known today. They had been very supportive of our programmes over the years. On several occasions we encountered problems, because at that time the area of mental health for people with ID was relatively unknown, and applications to mental health organisations for research funding were rejected on the grounds that it was not their remit. They suggested that we make applications to ID funding bodies, while

---

74 Holt G, Costello H, Bouras N, Diareme S, Hillery J, Moss S, Rodríguez Blázquez C, Salvador-Carulla L, Tsiantis J, Weber G & Dimitrakaki C (2000) BIOMED-MEROPE Project: service provision for adults with mental retardation: a European perspective. *Journal of Intellectual Disability Research* **44** 685–696.

conversely the latter were rejecting our applications as relevant not to them but to mental health!

In 2000 a very productive collaboration was established with Professor Peter Tyrer of Imperial College London. I had known Peter since my time at the MHAC (see also Chapter 2), when he had been in Nottingham during the early stages of community mental health developments. Peter is a very well-respected psychiatrist, both nationally and internationally, and has led many research projects. He is also a past editor of the *British Journal of Psychiatry*. Peter, in addition to community mental health, had a research interest in mental health and ID and had developed a collaboration with Professor Angela Hassiotis of the University College London. This probably followed a chance finding in the UK700 trial of intensive case management, where only people with borderline ID showed some improvement compared to those who received standard case management. As this finding was random and the group of people with borderline ID were possibly suffering with chronic schizophrenia, Peter Tyrer wanted to replicate this finding in a population of people with ID who were receiving ID services. Patricia Oliver-Africano was leading the research group in mental health in ID with Peter Tyrer, and at the Estia Centre we were trying to design a joint randomised controlled trial (RCT) to compare assertive community treatment with standard treatment. We ended up with two separate studies, one by Imperial College and the other by the Estia Centre, using a range of outcome measures. Neither study showed any major differences between the 'assertive' and 'standard' groups. In our study, we found no statistically significant differences between assertive and standard community treatments, in terms of the level of unmet needs, carer burden, functioning and quality of life, but we did find marginal evidence of a difference between treatment groups in terms of quality of life, and this was in favour of standard community treatment.[75]

We were successful in our collaboration with Peter Tyrer and in 2002 the Health Technology Assessment programme awarded us a major grant to carry out a randomised controlled trial (RCT) evaluating the effectiveness of antipsychotics compared to a placebo in treating people with ID and aggressive behaviour that was not due to psychotic illness. This was the first time that such an RCT was conducted. The project was led by Peter Tyrer in collaboration with the Estia Centre, as well as with Professors Declan Murphy, Shoumitro Deb and Martin Knapp. The project became known as NACHBID (Neuroleptics for Adults with Challenging Behaviour and Intellectual Disabilities), an acronym that I had suggested. The results did not show any benefit of risperidone and haloperidol compared with placebo in people with ID and aggressive behaviour. The first paper was published in the *Lancet* and attracted vast interest and publicity.[76] On reflection, however, I think that the outcomes of this trial were rather overplayed. Though the sample was adequate for statistical analysis, it was nevertheless relatively small and of low power. Most importantly, the sample was collected from several heterogeneous services and in small numbers. In our service, to our disappointment, we were not able to identify more than a small handful of people who fulfilled the inclusion criteria. This does not suggest that

75 Martin G, Costello H, Leese M, Slade M, Bouras N, Higgins S & Holt G (2005) An exploratory study of assertive community treatment for people with intellectual disability and psychiatric disorders: Conceptual, clinical, and service issues. *Journal of Intellectual Disability Research* **49** (7) 516–524.

76 Tyrer P, Oliver-Africano P, Ahmed Z, Bouras N, Cooray S, Deb S *et al* (2008) Risperidone, haloperidol and placebo in the treatment of aggressive challenging behaviour in patients with intellectual disability: A randomised controlled trial *The Lancet* **371** (9606) 57–63.

antipsychotics should be used in people with ID and aggressive behaviour, but that a replication of a similar study with a larger sample not drawn from several heterogeneous services as being designed currently, would be important.

Colin Hemmings has provided a critical overview of how the health service delivery research output from the Estia Centre evolved over a period of 25 years:

'The major strength of the research of the Estia Centre and the reason for its wider influence has been its strong focus on psychiatric disorders and challenging behaviours rather than on the primary health care or social care of people with ID. Primary health and social care service delivery to people with ID and the evaluation of it is also of critical importance, but it was recognized that specialist mental health services should focus on their core role and the ongoing development and improvement of expertise in this area. This recognition was not always shared by other ID services in the UK, particularly at the time of inception of the Estia Centre and its allied clinical service in South East London. Estia Centre encouraged a culture of research, locally, nationally and internationally. One of the strengths of the published research output was how it had often been linked in with several and substantial training initiatives as described above, conferences, texts for specialists and non-specialists and wider policy debates.' [77]

---

77 Hemmings C (2010) Service use and outcomes. In: N Bouras and G Holt (eds) *Mental Health Services for Adults with Intellectual Disability: Strategies and solutions*. Hove: Psychology Press.

A common peer reviewer criticism of the papers that we submitted for publication, was that our studies were restricted to our own sample of service users and had no wider application. With such a paucity of health service research in our field, we felt that this criticism was unjustified. We never claimed the generalisability of our health service research, but relied instead on thorough documentation of applied clinical practice. Inevitably, there were a number of limitations to the research of the Estia Centre. There were ongoing problems with recruitment of people with ID for research, and these were unfortunately exacerbated by the properly increased standards of ethical approval required to undertake research with vulnerable people, where capacity to consent to take part may often be impaired. Some of the studies have been retrospective, with the attendant potential for bias. It is also true that outcome measures used have not been as wide as it is currently recognised they should be. For example, it is now widely accepted that outcomes should include such measures as carer burden, service user satisfaction, quality of life and an economic evaluation of existing or new service delivery.

Despite this, Estia Centre research into health service delivery at least helped to provide the foundation to address the specialist versus generic services question. The context of this research work was the foresight and determination to evaluate from the outset of deinstitutionalisation what services were providing and what service users needed. The MHiLD staff in the 1980s, and later, those at the Estia Centre, showed great application in collecting data on their referrals ever since their inception of the services. From an early stage, they were committed to evidence-based practice. Owing to this vision and perceptiveness, the Estia Centre has provided a major contribution towards the rapid expansion of the evidence base in health service delivery for people with ID and mental health problems.

Clinical audit

The Estia Centre conducted or participated in a wide range of clinical audits, including the following:

- The Regional Audit of Low Secure Facilities for People with Learning Disabilities and Mental Disorder and Very Complex Needs was conducted in 2004 in collaboration with Oxleas NHS Trust. Of 200 inpatients in low secure units in the South East Thames Region, one-third were assumed to be in an inappropriate level of security, with most of these thought to require a lower level. For those in mental health units, being female and not being a risk to others predicted a need for a lower level of security. For those in ID units, being younger and admitted on an informal basis predicted a need for a lower level of security.

- The Regional Audit of the Care Programme Approach (CPA) and Risk Assessment/Management Implementation for Community Service Users with ID and Mental Health Problems, was carried out in 2002 and led by David Brooks. This audit found that there was limited implementation of CPA and other standards set out within the *National Service Framework for Mental health* relating to people with ID and mental health problems. Primary care trusts and community learning disability teams were less likely to implement the CPA and risk assessment/ management than specialist mental health of ID teams within mental health and ID trusts. There were few joint protocols between learning disability services and adult mental health, primary care and criminal justice systems.

- The Audit of Referrals of People with Borderline
  Cognitive Impairments in the Boroughs of Lambeth,
  Southwark and Lewisham in 2005 concluded that
  there was difficulty establishing and implementing
  uniform eligibility criteria across the service. Even
  when criteria were matched, it was not always
  possible to ascertain whether the impairments were
  developmental in origin. The results indicated a
  fragmented service configuration, a lack of clear
  clinical protocols and a need to develop more
  effective services for those falling within the upper
  margins of ID range.

- The Audit of the Quality of Follow-up Letters
  between GPs and MHiLD in 2006 showed that GPs
  were generally satisfied with the quality, timing and
  length of follow-up letters. All clinical items included
  in the letters were considered to be important and
  essential. Compared to other items, the Mental State
  Examination and Risk Assessment were viewed as
  less important. This was possibly because letters
  tended to be written for a wide range of professionals
  and therefore might contain information that was
  less important for some professionals than others.

These clinical audits were of major importance for
looking at the quality standards of organising and
delivering services.

Service user involvement

From its inception, the Estia Centre viewed service user
involvement as an integral part of its work. It regularly
consulted with service users and advocacy organisations
regarding service development and delivery. People with
ID were also involved in the development and delivery

of training initiatives and consulted on a number of research projects.

In 2004 the Estia Centre decided to make service user involvement one of its formal priorities, led by Steve Hardy and Eddie Chaplin and supported by a newly appointed service user development coordinator. The coordinator had a remit across SLaM, particularly within the Adults with Learning Disabilities Division, and worked closely with other local statutory service providers. Key stakeholders across Lambeth, Lewisham and Southwark were consulted on service user involvement, and several projects were instigated. A forum was developed for service users on the Weston Unit and one of the forum's first achievements was to produce a bill of rights for service users. The coordinator interviewed people with ID who were using our services regarding their satisfaction with their care. Other key areas were service user involvement in interview panels for psychology and nursing staff, and representation on local Learning Disability Partnership Boards. Another role of the coordinator was to liaise closely with other departments within SLaM, including complaints and clinical governance. An important part of service user involvement was the ongoing development of the Tuesday Group. This was a mental health promotion group for people with ID living in the London Borough of Lewisham. It was originally set up in 2001 as a 10-week course but owing to the positive evaluation it received and the need for ongoing support, the group continued indefinitely. The group originally met fortnightly at the local Mencap shop outside the Estia Centre campus, and members discussed how they could promote their own mental health. The group covered a variety of topics such as risk and protective factors, assertiveness skills, social skills, advocacy and understanding ones own emotions. The success and positive experiences in working with this group led to initiatives such as employing members of the group on an 'as required' basis for tasks such as service audits and consultation events. The Tuesday Group also presented at several national conferences on mental health and people with learning disabilities.

Mental Health in Learning Disabilities Nurses Forum

Nursing colleagues played a pivotal role in the continuing development of the Estia Centre activities. The objectives of the Estia Centre on nursing were mainly to assist in the implementation of SLaM's nursing strategy within the learning disability services. The Mental Health in Learning Disability Nurses Forum, set up in 2003 and led by Steve Hardy, worked admirably hard to promote the aims of the Estia Centre. The aim was to promote and develop nursing practice to meet the mental health needs of people with ID. The forum was free and open to any registered nurse from across the UK. The main objectives were to exchange knowledge and information, to explore and examine evidence-based practice, to develop a support network, to develop a competency framework for nurses working in the field, the professional development of nurses, and the development of mental health nursing care in learning disability as a sub-specialty of both mental health and learning disability nursing. The forum held four meetings a year. Each meeting concentrated on a particular issue that was decided by the forum's members. Topics included assessment, treatment and competencies for nurses, and service models. Members also had access to the Mental Health in Learning Disabilities Network. This was an email network that allowed members to share information and seek help and advice. The network also disseminated information and resources.

Consultancy

The Estia Centre was involved in offering advice and consultation to several service providers nationally and internationally. The integration of the clinical services with the Estia Centre, and the expertise of its members in developing and running services for people with ID and mental health problems and/or challenging behaviour needs, offered unique opportunities for sharing experience and knowledge with other services. Specially tailored packages were developed and these took into consideration diverse local needs. The Estia Centre was commissioned to undertake several reviews and evaluations of different services by the Estia Centre were commissioned nationally and internationally.

Visitors

The Estia Centre received a regular stream of visitors: professionals in mental health and ID, managers, policy makers etc. from across the UK and all over the world. These visitors came wanting to learn about and examine local service models and the interface between the clinical services and the Estia Centre. Some organisations also sent students for specially tailored educational and training programmes.

Today, the Estia Centre continues to offer its services and expertise with an expanded programme. This can be viewed at www.estiacentre.org

Chapter 11: The university component

The Section

It will already be clear that our activities over the years had a strong academic component. These academic activities were initially organised from the Section for the Psychiatry of Mental Handicap – renamed to Section for the Psychiatry of Learning Disabilities. The Section was created within the structure of the Academic Department of Psychiatry of UMDS at Guy's Hospital.[78]

The main aim of our Section was to promote teaching, training and R&D in services and clinically related areas in the field of ID. The members of the Section were all consultant psychiatrists working in MHiLD and associated services. Senior registrars/specialist registrars, clinical psychologists, nurses and other professionals working in ID joined the activities of the Section ad hoc or for specific projects.

---

78 The other Sections of the Academic Department of Psychiatry of UMDS were the Section of Old Age, chaired initially by Professor Elaine Murphy and then Professor Alastair McDonald; Community Psychiatry, chaired by Professor Tom Craig; Child and Adolescent, chaired initially by Professor Tony Cox and later by Professor Emily Simonoff; and Liaison Psychiatry, chaired by Professor Amanda Ramirez.

All were NHS employees and they used nominal academic time for the activities of the Section. There was no infrastructure in terms of offices, equipment, or administration provided by the university, and we did not receive any funds from the Higher Education Funding Council for England (HEFCE). All funds were raised either from NHS-related activities, or grants or fees from lectures and training. The Section was a very useful vehicle for carrying out academic activities that were almost entirely related to clinical matters and services, keeping colleagues up to date with research and developments, and at the same time giving them the opportunity to teach both undergraduate medical students and multidisciplinary postgraduate students at diploma and master's levels. At the same time, we had the flexibility to organise external seminars and conferences and develop training materials. I chaired the Section, as I was the only one who had a formal appointment with the university while being contractually an NHS employee.

Teaching and training occupied a major part of Section members' time. We organised the undergraduate teaching of medical students on mental health aspects of ID at UMDS. The teaching involved introductory and advanced lectures on mental health in ID. In addition, undergraduates attended outpatient clinics and community visits, and they were offered attachments to families with a member who had ID. Occasionally, students were attached to people with ID and complex mental health needs in order to act as their advocates, so they became familiar with ethical and legal issues involved in the care of this population.

Institute of Public Health South East Thames

In 1993 Dr Helen Mair, consultant in public health in South East Kent, approached me about developing the mental health services for people with ID in the Medway area. Helen was a formidable colleague who knew what she wanted and cared about high-quality services. Helen was also chairing the Institute of Public Health in South East Thames and set up a working party together with Ann Gath, then professor of ID at University College London and registrar of the Royal College of Psychiatrists, Geraldine Holt, and me to address the mental health needs of People with ID in the South East Thames region. The publication of the report of the working party was well received by the regional officers and was favourably reviewed by Professor Bill Fraser.[79] This resulted in Helen being able to create an NHS consultant post in ID in Medway with two days academic work at the UMDS at Guy's. At the time, this sort of NHS consultant post was encouraged, in order to attract high-quality candidates. Dr Sabah Sadik was appointed to that post and moved from Liverpool, where he was already consultant, to Medway, and he became senior lecturer in the Section. Sabah became an integrated member of the Section and worked closely with us until he took a sabbatical and then left his post.

Research and Development

Research was also a major part of the activities of the Section. When the Estia Centre was established in

79 Fraser WI (1993) The mental health needs of people with learning disability. *Psychiatric Bulletin* **18** 122–126.

1999 all of the activities of the Section were undertaken operationally from the Estia Centre and these are described in more detail in Chapter 10. In essence, the Estia Centre became the Section, although we also formally kept the Section structure within the academic department.

Mental Health Studies Programme (MSc)

A few months before his retirement in 2000, Professor Jim Watson invited me to take over the chair of the Mental Health Studies Programme. I accepted this challenge and was fully aware of the enormity of the task. I was taking over what had been one of Jim's many successful initiatives as chairman of the Division of Psychiatry and Psychology at Guy's.

The Mental Health Studies Programme, known as 'MSc', was established in 1990 by Professor Jim Watson. The aim was to provide high-quality, up-to-date coverage of theory, practice and research in mental health and psychiatric illness. It was designed primarily for students who already had some experience of working in the mental health field – in clinical, therapeutic or educational capacities – and who wanted to build on their existing knowledge, experience and understanding. All the courses in the programme were taught by staff who reflected the multidisciplinary ethos of the programme; they were drawn from psychiatry, nursing, psychotherapy, psychology, social work, occupational therapy, and so on. Most units had regular contributions from practising clinicians and visiting lecturers who were specialists in their fields. Because much of the learning and teaching took place in groups of no more than 20 students, sessions were typically interactive and students' contributions were encouraged. Each year there was a series of occasional Saturday research workshops. These were designed to introduce students to the principles of research and to provide the foundations for their own research projects. While there were a small number of students who were full-time, the vast majority of students on the programme were part-time, completing the master's courses in two years and the postgraduate diploma courses in one year.

The MSc Mental Health Studies consisted of three units: a compulsory basic mental health unit and two elective units. The basic unit provided an overview of theoretical perspectives on psychiatric illness, diagnosis and assessment, psychiatric disorders, and treatment. Students were offered the opportunity to pursue their interests and to develop more in-depth knowledge and understanding of particular aspects of mental health and illness through the two elective units. These elective units included anthropology, cognitive analytic therapy, cognitive-behavioural therapy, community psychiatry, dynamic psychotherapy, eating disorders, forensic psychiatry, inpatient/Psychiatric Intensive Care Unity (PICU) care, learning disabilities, management, motivational interviewing, organisational psychiatry and psychology, research, and women's mental health.

Since its inception in the early 1990s, the MSc had grown into a postgraduate programme with a yearly intake of approximately 100 students. The majority of these worked in the NHS and were registered as part-time students. When the fifteenth anniversary of the programme was celebrated at Guy's on 23 May 2006, more than 600 people had graduated with an MSc in Mental Health Studies or one of its related programmes.

Several colleagues from the Division of Psychiatry and Psychology at Guy's and the extended associate department were involved with the running and teaching

of the MSc. When I took it over in 2000, the merger of
the Division of Psychiatry at Guy's and St Thomas' with
the Division of Psychological Medicine at the Institute
of Psychiatry was underway. This was a very complex
task involving several issues that had to be disentangled.
The MSc then came under the quality assurance process
of King's College London (KCL) and had to deal with
a phenomenal amount of bureaucracy, to which Jim
Watson had always been averse. It should be pointed
out that the MSc was a significant income generator for
the division perhaps of several multiplies of the R&D
grants then obtainable by other academic departments.
At that time, the Division of Psychological Medicine at
the IoP was research-oriented and had little experience
and no significant interest in taught courses. However,
the income generated by the MSc was very attractive!
At the same time, KCL wanted to maximise its share of
income and for no clear reason had budgeted the MSc
wrongly. There were several bureaucratic problems,
with several departments involved, and some very time-
consuming meetings that were not all pleasant. I felt
that for a major educational institution to have such a
lack of vision and direction in such an important area
of teaching was beyond belief.

With the help of Tom Craig and Jed Boardman,
we managed to sort out the basic difficulties and
problems. We were helped decisively by Karen Baistow,
whom we appointed as programme director for the MSc.
The whole programme was reviewed and eventually
comprised of the following components: MSc Mental
Health Studies, MSc Organisational Psychiatry
and Psychology, MSc in Addiction Counselling, MSc
Mental Health in Learning Disabilities (LD), and
MSc in Clinical Psychotherapy of Cognitive Analytic
Psychotherapy. (The MSc Mental Health in Learning
Disabilities is described in Chapter 10 about the

Estia Centre, as it was delivered from there.)

In the meantime, radical changes were taking place in academia, including academic psychiatry. Appraisals and evaluations were introduced, outputs were measured in detail and there was a climate fully alien to the one we had worked so hard to create at Guy's and St Thomas'. When Jim Watson retired at the end of 2000, there were 20 colleague psychiatrists, psychologists and nurses from our academic department of psychiatry who had been awarded a professorship and had been working in various prestigious academic establishments. There were also numerous others had been awarded senior lectureships. The psychiatric rotational training scheme had been expanded to include training posts in Kent and Sussex, and most of the psychiatric services in the South East Thames region were staffed by ex-Guy's trainees who became consultant psychiatrists and had contributed significantly to raising the standards and quality of care of psychiatric patients.

The Diploma of Psychiatric Practice (DPP) was another training innovation of the Academic Department of Psychiatry at Guy's that was initiated by Jim Watson. The DPP was established as a joint diploma by the Academic Department of Psychiatry of UMDS with colleagues at the Institute of Psychiatry of the Ain Shams University in Cairo. A joint task force developed the course and the examinations procedures. The deans of the two medical schools had signed a resultant agreement between the two institutions. The first diplomas were awarded in 1995, and between then and 2002 a total of 172 diplomas were awarded. The key features of this diploma programme were that students should be taught the psychiatry they would actually need in their country of practice and that they must be examined in the language in which they would actually practice, as they were not going to work in NHS psychiatry and systems. A key feature of the agreement with Ain Shams was that it allowed us to set fees to cover the courses and diploma that were reasonable for those from low-income countries – something that UK regulations did not allow.

Later, the Department of Psychiatry of the Fountain House Network in Lahore, Pakistan also joined the programme. The concept was to provide mental health professionals with knowledge and skills necessary to deliver efficient psychiatric service in primary care and community settings, paying due attention to local, social and cultural circumstances. The syllabus generally included eight modules, such as dynamic psychopathology, psychiatric classification and diagnosis, interviewing examination and basement, psychiatric treatment, the cultural context of psychiatric disorders, service planning and administration, service monitoring and evaluation, and the psychiatrist and the mental health team. Although much of the actual day-to-day teaching was carried out by academics abroad, the curriculum was devised by the academic staff at Guy's, who had control of the standards of the course and the examinations. The DPP was popular mostly in Arab countries, and certainly provided a basic training for general practitioners and psychiatrists practising in these countries at a time when only limited training and exposure to modern aspects of psychiatry were provided elsewhere. The DPP was an important activity of the Academic Department of Psychiatry at Guy's; several colleagues visited Ain Shams University in Cairo and the department in London likewise received many colleagues from Ain Shams. Every effort was made to maintain the highest standards for the course. When UMDS merged with KCL, the latter did not recognised the DPP and forced us to suspend it. The intake of students was suspended in 2001 and I had to travel to Cairo on Christmas day in 2002 to examine the last DPP students who were still in the system.

After discussions with colleagues in Ain Shams we decided to take forward this concept of training and to widen the opportunities for more people in more countries, by making it possible to study for the DPP by distance learning. The application submitted for approval to the Teaching and Learning Committee of the IoP was sadly not approved and the DPP was ceased. Some planned later efforts to revive it did not materialise.

I handed over the chair of the MSc to Dr Sukhi Shergill of the Division of Psychological Medicine at the IoP at the end of 2006.[80] The transition was very smooth and Sukhi took over the responsibility of running the programme with interest and curiosity. It was a pleasure to work with Sukhi during the transition period. The MSc was reorganised and continues to flourish today. It makes a substantial financial contribution to the IoP and KCL, and this was eventually recognised. Two annual prizes were established by my successors. These were named after Jim Watson and myself, and both of us have been invited regularly to the prize-giving event before Christmas each year.

The mergers

The academic department went through a long transition period during the anticipated merger of UMDS with KCL, which was officially agreed in 1998.

---

80 At that time, the programme included three MScs: Mental Health Studies, Organisational Psychiatry and Psychology, and Mental Health in Learning Disabilities. Karen Baistow was leading Mental Health Studies, Gilly Wiscarson led Organisational Psychiatry and Psychology, and Elias Tsakanikos led Mental Health in Learning Disabilities.

Following the merger the Academic Department of Psychiatry came under Guy's, King's, St Thomas' Medical School (GKT) of King's College London (KCL). With this structure there were, however, two Divisions of Psychiatry within GKT: the Division of Psychiatry and Psychology at Guy's, with Jim Watson as chairman, and the Division of Psychological Medicine at the IoP, with Professor Robin Murray as chairman. Long-lasting discussions soon started about the future of the two academic departments. These discussions had to deal with the additional complication that the two Divisions of Psychiatry had different orientations, cultures and ethoses. The Guy's division was focused on teaching, learning and training, and clinically oriented research related to mental health services. There was at Guy's a shared democratic working atmosphere among colleagues, who were committed to development and provision of high-quality mental health services. The IoP division was oriented towards mostly biological and epidemiological research, with limited teaching and learning involvement. Furthermore, there was pressure from the implications of the Research Assessment Exercise (RAE) in 1999 related to the funding of the academic departments. The decision was made for the two divisions to merge in 1999 and as Jim Watson was about to retire the following year, Robin Murray became the chairman of the new joint Division of Psychological Medicine and Tom Craig became vice-chairman, being accountable to the Deans of GKT and IoP. In practice, this merger was implemented in 2002.

In 2000 a series of valedictory lectures at Guy's, St Thomas' and IoP was organised to mark the retirement of Jim Watson. The series, which was entitled 'Reflections: 1974 to 2000', included five lectures:

- 'What does, and what should, the clinical academic psychiatrist do?'
  – Guy's Hospital, January 2000.

- 'Illness behaviour and help-seeking' – St Thomas' Hospital, February 2000.

- 'Individual approaches to psychopathology and psychological treatments'
  – Institute of Psychiatry, March 2000.

- 'Couples sexuality and relationships' – Guy's Hospital, September 2000.

- 'Groups, communities and the inpatient environment' – St Thomas' Hospital, October 2000.

Finally, the valedictory conference, entitled 'From Theory to Practice in Academic Psychiatry', took place at Guy's on 1 December 2000. I was privileged to chair this event. It offered a very rich programme that included talks on:

- 'Doctors and sex in 1990', by Dominic Beer and Andrew Hodgkiss

- 'Psychospiritosexobiosocio self-status and psychiatric practice in Bermondsey' by Kam Buhi

- 'Applying psychological practice to psychiatric practice', by Anthony Ryle

- 'The social origins of depression', by George Brown and Tyrril Harris

- 'How to garage your study', by Stan Newman

- 'Naturalistic nations and NICE nonsense in psychiatry', by Tony Hale

- 'The talking cure', by Derry Macdiarmid

- 'The vice president and the brigadier', by Lawrence Meassey

- 'Jim Watson and Ireland', by Anthony McCarthy

- 'Jim's Community', by Tom Craig

- 'Psychology and management', by Isobel Morris

- 'Education for all: the MSc in mental health studies', by James Lindesay

- 'Wake up! And get off the chair', by Bob Jezzard

- 'Military, managerial and academic (in)competence', by Jim Watson.

It was a memorable day that was very much in the spirit and style of Jim Watson. The conference was attended by over 200 people who had at different times been associated with the Academic Department of Psychiatry. Several people had worked hard in organising this event, but it was mostly our dedicated and most helpful administrators and personal assistants (PAs), as they were called at that time; Kay Scutt of the Academic Department and Chris Thomas of the York Clinic, who did the bulk of the organising. It was a moving occasion at which we paid tribute to Jim Watson, a charismatic colleague and major contributor to modern British psychiatry and beyond.

Needless to say that all the processes associated with the merger over the years were very confusing to several of us, and on a personal level I felt I had lost my direction! The new Division of Psychological Medicine was the largest in Europe, and probably in the world, as it brought together 300 clinicians, researchers and teachers at the forefront of research into many aspects of psychiatry. Many members of the division worked as psychiatrists and psychologists within SLaM. The undergraduate teaching, led by Tief Davis, and the basic and specialist postgraduate training was brought under the management of the new division. The same applied to research and a new strategy was developed that structured research into different Interdisciplinary Research Groups (IRGs).

Those of us coming from GKT were free to choose whether we would be under the new Division of Psychological Medicine or not and were also able to sit under two academic departments at the IoP. Some time prior to this, Graham Thornicroft, whom I had known as a medical student at Guy's and at the time of the MHAC, had begun a very important and exciting development at the IoP: the Health Service Research Department, today known as Health Service and Population Research Department (HSPRD). The HSPRD was situated in a new modern building on the IoP campus, which was named the David Goldberg Centre in recognition of Professor Sir David Goldberg's immense contribution to psychiatry worldwide. This department was closer to my research interests, as it had sections on community psychiatry, primary care, mental health economics, psychiatric nursing, cultural psychiatry, mental health and aging, quality and clinical governance, sociomedical research, social work, rehabilitation in severe psychosis, as well as a World Health Organization (WHO) collaborating centre and later global mental health. David Goldberg was very actively involved in setting up the HSPRD, as were professors Antony Mann, George Szmukler, Martin Prince, Martin Knap, Andree Tylee, Dinesh Bhugra, Mike Slade, Kevin Gourney and others.

I had a dilemma as to which department I should choose to join, as I had the responsibility for the MSc at Guy's and the Estia Centre. There was also strong interest from both academic departments, primarily because of the income generated by the MSc. Eventually, following agonising discussions with Tom Craig, we decided that the MSc would sit in the new Division of Psychiatry on moral grounds, as it was a venture of the Guy's Division of Psychiatry, and we as individuals should join both HSPRD and Psychological Medicine. In the subsequent years I always felt that I belonged to HSPRD, and Graham Thornicroft and other colleagues there were very supportive of me and the Estia Centre. There was an attempt in 2005 with the HSPRD to develop a chair in the psychology of ID that would be strongly linked with the Estia Centre, but this did not materialise owing to restrictions on new academic appointments and the RAE.

Janet Treasure took over as chair of psychiatry at Guy's, but in a short time, following more structural changes, there was no academic department of Psychiatry at Guy's; in a few years, there was not even a clinical department. Even the historic York Clinic closed and all inpatient psychiatric services were moved to the Maudsley Hospital. It seemed a very backward step, after fighting for many years to have psychiatric departments within general hospitals, to abandon them and return to having separate mental hospitals. It was also terribly heartbreaking after all the efforts we had made over so many years to raise the standards of psychiatry based at Guy's, under the inspirational leadership of Jim Watson, and the innovations we had ushered in in teaching, training, research and services. There was a time during Margaret Thatcher's NHS reforms in the late 1980s that the Maudsley Hospital, as a special health authority with a small catchment area, was seriously threatened, while Guy's, having joined Lewisham and with its large catchment area, seemed secure. It is now history that Guy's psychiatry was absorbed by the Maudsley instead of the other way round, as seemed more likely at that time of past reforms.

Chapter 12: The international dimension

California

In 1984, while our plans for the closure of Darenth Park and the reprovision of services were shaping up, and the development of community services and community mental handicap teams were gradually being put in place, I had an unexpected proposal. Angela Summerfield, of the Department of Social Psychology at Birkbeck College, London University (who was also working in our Academic Department of Psychiatry), had agreed with Paul Ekman for him to be a visiting professor in London for three months. Paul Ekman was an eminent and world-renowned professor of social psychology at University of California, San Francisco. His latest book at that time, *Telling Lies*, described his research on recognising lies from people's facial expressions. It was a bestseller and had attracted wide interest from the scientific community, as well as governmental offices and services such as the police and the courts. Paul would come to London only on the condition that he could exchange houses with someone there, as he was coming with his wife and his two children. The Ekmans' house was situated in Berkley Hills in San Francisco. Jim Watson suggested that the

Ekmans might exchange their house in San Francisco with my family's home in Blackheath, as this would give me an opportunity to look at the US services and programmes in psychiatry and ID. Jim covered my clinical duties with the help of Geraldine Holt, who had started her training with us as senior registrar a few months earlier.

I was granted three months leave of absence and in early September 1985 I arrived with my wife Maria and my daughters Christine and Irene at the Ekmans' house in Berkley (with its panoramic view of the Bay area), while Paul Ekman arrived with his wife Mary Ann Mason and their son Tom and daughter Eva at our house in Blackheath. That was the only kind of sabbatical that I ever took over my 35 years' service in the NHS and the university. A lot of preparation had taken place for this visit and Paul Ekman had visited us to inspect our house and make all sort of practical arrangements such as finding schools for the children. This was a most enjoyable life experience for both of our families and since then my wife and I have developed a long-lasting friendship with Paul and Mary Ann Ekman. We have exchanged houses for holidays a few more times since then, with us staying at their new houses (always with magnificent views) in Twin Peaks and Embarcadero in San Francisco, and the Ekmans staying at our new house in London.

Paul made available to me his office at the University of California, San Francisco (UCSF), in Parnassus Avenue, and introduced me to several of his colleagues. California had advanced community-based services for people with ID. There were, however, still some very large institutions in the San Francisco area, in the Napa Valley and Sonoma, as well as in Los Angeles. I visited several services, including institutions and community services, and met many people while I attended a series of planning and information meetings in Sacramento, the capital of California, where the Health Administration headquarters were based. Interestingly, most of the meetings took place at hotels near airports, so that people could easily fly in and out from other cities and states.

The process of closing the Californian institutions had slowed down, and in some areas had almost ceased, while in the UK it was about to gain momentum. There were well-developed community services in the form of developmental disabilities centres (a term adopted in California), which offered assessment and consultation mainly to people with ID, but also to those with autistic spectrum disorders, epilepsy and some physical disabilities. There was no separation of health and social services. Providers called vendors were contracted for residential, day care and other services on an annual basis. Mental health care was not provided or contracted by the developmental disabilities centres, and that was a major problem. Generic psychiatric services were refusing to serve people with ID on the grounds that the predominant problem was not psychiatric and they were not contracted and had no expertise to support a group of people with highly individual needs – a well-known problem in the UK, which has already been described several times in this book. Most of the people I met were public administrators, clinical psychologists, nurses and social workers. They were surprised to hear that I was a psychiatrist involved with the development of community services for people with ID, as because of the funding systems in the US, psychiatry was separated from ID services.

One very interesting experience was my visit to the University of California in Los Angeles (UCLA), which in the early 1960s was the first university in the country to be awarded federal support for both a university-affiliated and its companion programme, and the

Mental Retardation Research Centre. The two operated with a unified administration in the Neuropsychiatric Institute, part of the UCLA Centre for Health Services. Peter Tanguy, the director of the programme, described to me the provision of the programme's high standard of developmental disabilities training for professionals in administration, community liaison, nursing, special education, child psychiatry, etc. The Mental Retardation Research Centre conducted several research projects for the study of early childhood psychosis. A clinical inpatient and outpatient service at UCLA was also offered to developmentally disabled people suffering from psychiatric problems.

The developmental disabilities services in California were characterised by clarity of operational roles with legislative cover, one integrated health and social services state provider, accountability, flexibility and relatively adequate financial provision. Californian developmental disabilities services had a very impressive computerised data information system available for both service delivery and planning purposes. The main problems they experienced were the increasingly high cost of purchasing programmes and services from vendors, especially for people with both developmental disabilities and psychiatric disorders. The two services for mental retardation and mental health were separated, and no provision was made for those people who would need both of them. There was a tendency for each service to consider the other one to be responsible and, as a consequence, people might receive service from neither. Developmental disabilities services believed that their service users should have access to generic services, including for mental health. But psychiatric services argued that most of the symptoms manifested by these service users were due to their mental retardation and not to treatable psychiatric disorders. Such demarcation disputes were only too familiar in the UK. A 'task force' had been formed in California by interested parties to study the problems and propose action. In spite of two years' work, the study had not been completed, and the provision of beds for crises admissions presented continuing problems. Local arrangements known as 'interim working agreements' were in force in some places and these relieved some of the pressure temporarily. Psychiatrists were reluctant to attend non-medical facilities or go on domiciliary visits, as they were not reimbursed by the complicated medical insurance system. These problems created various obstacles in the US system, and the NHS was undoubtedly superior in this respect, in terms of making it easier for doctors to work in community settings. Some other long-term planning problems for California included the impact on services when all people eligible for service had been identified and the increasing ageing population with developmental disabilities.

I also had the opportunity to look at the general psychiatric services in San Francisco. These had run into major problems, with people with psychiatric disorders being lost in the streets of San Francisco and other large cities. There was a climate of despair among clinicians and managers, and an overall impression that the community care plans of the 1960s had failed. Community care for people with mental health problems had not even started yet in the UK, except for some early initiatives such as the MHAC in Lewisham (see Chapter 2). When I mentioned to American colleagues our plans to move rapidly to community care, they all unanimously responded, 'Don't!' Obviously, our mental health systems were different, and I believe that we fared better in the UK with our planned re-provision of services than in the US. I described my experiences and impressions from the California visit in an article

published in the *Psychiatric Bulletin*.[81] This visit to
California was very helpful for me and prepared me
to face the issues back home with open eyes and more
confidence as to what needed to be done.

Dual Diagnosis Conference, Chicago

A year later, in 1986, I was invited to a conference
in Chicago on dual diagnosis: the concept that, in
some people, both conditions of ID and mental health
problems can coexist and it is wrong to talk about
either of them separately. All the known Americans in
the field were in Chicago. These included Steve Reiss,
clinical psychologist, who was the first to start specialist
outpatient services for people with dual diagnosis in the
US; Johnny Matson, also a clinical psychologist, who
pioneered the early research in dual diagnosis; Ludwik
Szymanski, a child psychiatrist from Boston with a
special interest in autism; and Frank Menolascino, a
psychiatrist from Nebraska who pioneered the ENCOR
'core and cluster' model and was a very strong advocate
of community care.

Nebraska

Frank Menolascino had become the leading figure
in dual diagnosis and, in fact, he was the one who
introduced the concept, which was later adopted by the
substance misuse services. Frank had served in the US
President's Committee on Mental Retardation and the
National Institute of Mental Health. He was also the
recipient of the Outstanding Psychiatrist in America

---

81 Bouras N (1987) Developmental disabilities service in California.
Bulletin of the Royal College of Psychiatrists **11** 8–10.

award, a major outstanding achievement award presented by the American Psychiatric Association. Frank was an impressive charismatic personality of Italian American descent. He had a ready sense of humour and was quick with repartee. Frank had a background in adult community psychiatry, like me, and had been attracted by the ideas of normalisation theory and closing the institutions. I met Frank Menolascino again in 1989 at the World Psychiatric Association Congress in Athens and we started a collaboration that continued, together with a friendship, until his premature death in 1992.

In January 1990 Frank was invited by the Section of Mental Handicap of the Royal College of Psychiatrists to give the Blake Marsh lecture, which was one of the most prestigious annual events of the Section.[82] Frank gave an inspirational talk about the ENCOR project in Nebraska, the principles of community care and the closure of the institutions. Frank's talk was received with reservations by colleagues in London, who had expected a more 'scientific style' lecture based on empirical research, which was very limited at the time, while the scepticism about community care was high. The Blake Marsh lecture received a similar reaction in February 1994, when it was delivered by another American leader in the field of ID, the child psychiatrist Ludwik Szymanski from Harvard. The US and UK certainly took very different approaches to providing services for people with ID in the 1990s.

Frank invited me to visit the services in Omaha Nebraska in late 1990. This was another exciting experience as I was able to look at the ENCOR programme in person and talk to its main protagonists. Frank was very hospitable and I found him waiting for me with his

82 Day K & Jancar J (1997) Dr Blake Marsh and the Blake Marsh Lectures. *Psychiatric Bulletin* **21** 26–29.

wife Dona at the frozen Omaha airport in the middle of December. They both made my stay there very comfortable and enjoyable by organising several visits and meetings. Frank had brought to Nebraska Woolf Wolfensberger, the influential advocate of normalisation theory and later social valorisation (see also Chapter 5), as well as Bob Shallock, who developed the measurements of quality of life for people with ID. John McGee, the advocate of the 'gentle teaching approach', was also there. The community-based services that they had developed in Nebraska were impressive. This should be seen in the context of different service systems. Nebraska is a US agricultural state with vast countryside areas, very different from the inner-city areas of South East London. Frank was also chairman of the Academic Department of Psychiatry at Creighton University Medical School. Frank had supported the community care reforms with a strong mental health service, which included an inpatient specialist unit, within his general psychiatry services. ENCOR provided services to people with ID in the Eastern Nebraska Region. These included high-quality residential facilities in small houses and, most importantly, work experience through supported employment schemes in different businesses, such as in hotels, catering services and small manufacturing corporations.

I gave a series of lectures during my visit to Nebraska, including a grand round, where I presented our experience of developing community services in South East London, based on the closure of Darenth Park. The emphasis was on our specialist psychiatric model, as a 'bridge service between ID and mental health', opening a vigorous debate about the future of community-based services and the necessary psychiatric support.

ENCOR was conceived in 1970 as a comprehensive service system, with the parents' group assuming advisory and advocacy responsibility and remaining involved through the years, and notably during the expansion of the programme across Eastern Nebraska. ENCOR had attracted much interest internationally, and in fact this model was suggested by the Guy's 'Orange Report' (see Chapters 3 and 4), though it was later dropped for the model of 'ordinary housing' services. ENCOR had been visited by a UK Parliamentary Group, led by the Labour MP Rene Short, in 1981 and a report had been produced by Dr Lorna Wing of the Maudsley Hospital, a world-renowned psychiatrist in autism and ID (and wife of John Wing, professor of social psychiatry at the Maudsley Hospital and the IoP, a pioneer and world-recognised leader in social and community psychiatry in the 1970s and '80s). Lorna was known for her reservations about community care for people with ID and in her report from her visit to ENCOR, she concluded:

'I have no doubt that, even given equally good staff ratios and supervision to ensure 'quality control', smaller living groups offer markedly better care and opportunities for improvement than do the larger groups found in most mental handicap hospitals. Two questions remain unanswered for the independent observer. First, would a sheltered 'village' community with small living units have advantages for some retarded people, combining supervision and structure with more personal freedom than could be allowed for them in a normal community? Second, would a service like ENCOR, if it were set up in the UK, be able to cope with all the people with disturbed behaviour without costing considerably more than the State institutions and perhaps provoking adverse reactions from the community?'

Community care for all people with ID was a 'one-way street' and there was no return. Despite the fact that over three decades later, some of Lorna's points might still be valid – particularly those referring to people with problem (challenging) behaviour – other concerns have proved unfounded. For instance, local communities were overall accepting of people with ID in their neighbourhoods and nowadays this is normality. Lorna had personal experience through her daughter Susie, who had an autistic spectrum disorder. Lorna's contribution to the field was immense, as she initiated the Camberwell Case Register to record all people using psychiatric services in this area of South East London. Lorna was among the founders of the National Autistic Society and introduced the term Asperger's syndrome. I had the opportunity to collaborate with Lorna on several occasions, and I took a modest approach to her serious criticism about the way community care plans were implemented – which was not always unjustified! After her retirement from the Maudsley she was involved with the Centre for Social and Communication Disorders, the first integrated diagnostic and advice service for autistic spectrum disorders in the UK.

NADD

From Nebraska, I travelled together with Frank Menolascino to Boston for the seventh annual conference of what was known then as the National Association for the Dually Diagnosed (NADD), later renamed the National Association for Persons with Developmental Disabilities and Mental Health Needs. The evening before the conference we had a very pleasant meal in an Italian restaurant in Water Town in Boston together with Ludwik Szymanski and Louis

Fussaro, a clinical psychologist and NADD board member. As happens often in similar circumstances, we had a most interesting discussion covering many professional issues.

NADD was founded in 1983 as a not-for-profit association. The founder was Robert Fletcher, who is still the executive director of the organisation, and through his vision and leadership he has steered NADD to international prominence as a leading force in mental health for people with ID. The NADD conference was impressive and focused on mental health issues, instead of covering the wide range of issues in the field of ID. Frank was one of the keynote speakers and he articulated very clearly the existing gaps in the diagnosis, treatment and services for people with mental health problems and ID. Another impressive speaker was Robert Sovner, a psychiatrist specialising in mental health for people with ID in the Boston area. He carried out some of the early research in the field and also published a very interesting journal in a bulletin format, which was entitled *Mental Health Aspects of Developmental Disabilities*. Unfortunately, Robert Sovner died young. The publication of the journal was taken over for several years by Ann Hurley, psychologist, and Andrew Levitas, psychiatrist, both of whom are well known in the USA and abroad.

It was at that conference in Boston that I acquainted myself with several other American colleagues, in addition to those mentioned above, and began a collaboration with NADD that continued for many years. In 1995 NADD co-organised with the European Association for Mental Health in Mental Retardation (renamed the European Association of Mental Health in Intellectual Disabilities) the second International Conference in Mental Health and ID. I was an invited speaker at several NADD national and international conferences, and in 1995 I delivered the first Frank J.

Menolascino Lecture, at the International Congress
II, co-sponsored by NADD, Tufts University School of
Medicine and the European Association. The lecture
was entitled 'Dual Diagnosis towards the Year 2000'.
The emphasis of the Frank Menolascino lecture was
on the need for high-standard research in the field,
effective translation of research into practice, systematic
training for professionals but also for direct care staff,
and quality assurance as a necessary component at all
levels of service for people with mental health problems
and ID.

International Association for the Scientific Study of Intellectual and Develpmental Disabilities (IASSIDD)

In 1992 Ken Day and Jose Jancar nominated me to
join the Council of the IASSIDD, which was a well-
established international organisation for people with
ID and their families. It covered the broad spectrum
of issues relating to these groups, but without a
focus on mental health. The aim of IASSIDD was to
promote educational purposes and the scientific study
of intellectual disabilities and related developmental
disabilities worldwide. IASSIDD had been holding large
world congresses around the globe, which were attended
by a few thousand participants.

With Steve Moss, I convened an IASSIDD Special
Interest Research Group in Mental Health (SIRG-MH)
at a meeting at the Royal College of Psychiatrists in
London in 1995. The SIRG-MH was officially launched
at the Tenth IASSIDD World Congress in Helsinki

in 1996, where we organised 14 symposia on mental health topics. The first business meeting was attended by 73 colleagues, who endorsed the aims of the SIRG in mental health. The basic aim was to provide a focus for the worldwide exchange and dissemination of research and practice in the field of mental health of people with ID. Mental health was meant in the broadest sense, encompassing the full range of psychiatric, emotional and behavioural aspects. A wide variety of professional groups were potential contributors and no specific group was considered to have predominance in this respect. The SIRG also strived to promote cross-national, multidisciplinary collaboration in ID and mental health, and to provide a framework for the collation of information related to the research interests, expertise and publications of group members. In addition, within the overall process of collaboration, the views and contributions of non-professionals, including the people with intellectual disability themselves, and their families and friends, were a fundamental component, and would be given the priority they deserved. An ultimate aim of the SIRG's endeavours was to improve the quality of services for people with intellectual disability and their carers.[83]

The SIRG-MH organised two round tables in 1997: in Montreal in April, as part of the NADD International Conference, and in New York City in May, as part of the AAMR National Convention. A third round table took place in 1998 in Cambridge, UK. That was the first joint round table with SIRG-Aging. Another round table was organised in 1999 in London as part

83 For the history the following people had agreed to co-ordinate the activities of the SIRG in Mental Health until the next IASSIDD Congress XI in Seattle: John Hillery (Ireland), Dorothy Griffiths (Canada), Carina Gustafsson (Sweden), John Jacobson (USA), Steve Moss (UK), Bruce Tonge (Australia), Akihito Takahashi (Japan), Germain Weber (Austria) and Nick Bouras (UK).

of the Second European Congress of Mental Health in Mental Retardation. The format of the round tables was introduced by Matt Janicki, who specialised in ageing and ID. Matt played a fundamental role in IASSIDD and was an excellent organiser. I collaborated with him very productively on several international events over the years. We were trying to hold the round tables as part of other major conferences for practical reasons, and to avoid unnecessary duplications and financial risks. At that time, there was a proliferation of congresses, meetings and conferences in all fields, including mental health, being organised by several professional organisations and groups. With the increased financial cost and the continuing reduction of research funds, attendance at all these activities started becoming a problem. In September 1999 Tony Holland and John Jacobson took over the coordination of the SIRG-MH. John Jacobson (who also died young) was a serious thinker and researcher in both ID and mental health. We had a very fruitful collaboration that was documented in several publications.

I participated and contributed to the programme of the Eleventh IASSIDD Congress in Seattle in 2000 and the XII in Montpellier in 2004, both of which were very successful and included several symposia and presentations on the mental health aspects of people with ID. During my time with the IASSIDD, I had the opportunity to meet and work together with several esteemed colleagues, in addition to those referred to above. These included Phil Davidson and his colleague Nancy Cain from the Strong Centre in New York State, with whom we developed strong professional links, in association with the Estia Centre. Others included Stephen Kealy, Michael Mulcahy, Trevor Parmenter and Neil Ross. Montpellier was the last IASSIDD World Congress that I attended, and, having been vice president since 2000, I left the council as my term expired. I was awarded an honorary fellowship in 1999.

The council meetings of IASSIDD were interesting and informative. In one of them, which took place in Dublin in 1993, we were invited to a reception being held by Mrs Jean Kennedy-Smith, then the US Ambassadress to Ireland under President Clinton's administration. This had been arranged by the then president of IASSIDD, Terence Dolan of the Waisman Center at the University of Wisconsin–Madison. Mrs Jean Kennedy-Smith was sister to President John F. Kennedy, Senator Robert Kennedy and Rosemary Kennedy who, as explained in Chapter 3, was institutionalised in Wisconsin. At the time of our visit to Mrs Smith, her sister Patricia Kennedy-Lawford was also present, and when my Greek origin became known to the pair, the discussion was extended and dominated by comments about Jackie Kennedy-Onassis!

World Psychiatric Association (WPA)

I had been following the World Psychiatric Association's activities almost since I arrived in Britain in 1974. At that time, Dr Denis Leigh, consultant psychiatrist at the Maudsley Hospital, had organised a one-day WPA seminar in London at the Institute of Architects. This was a high-quality event with distinguished speakers including my trainer from Athens, Professor George Christodoulou. There were plenary presentations on new research and thorough reviews on clinical topics in psychiatry. I attended the Seventh WPA World Congress in Vienna in 1983 and gave several presentations on the latest findings from the ward environment research. With Hilary Standish-Barry and Paul Bridges, we presented the use of trazodone in depression, and with Douglas Brough and Jim Watson, we presented the Mental Health Advice Centre (MHAC) in Lewisham. The talk about the MHAC was received with scepticism by the audience. Community psychiatry was still in its very early stages, and the reports from the US were not very favourable. Douglas Brough had little experience of international conferences and the great diversity in the quality of presentations rather surprised him. This was exaggerated by the rather cool reception he received on the development of the MHAC, a topic we ourselves believed to be great importance for the future of psychiatric services.

The next WPA World Congress VIII took place in Athens in 1999. It was organised by Professor Costas Stefanis, of Athens University Medical School, who had been elected president of the WPA at the previous congress in Vienna. At that time, there was an explosive climate within the WPA, fuelled by the expulsion of the Soviet Union Psychiatric Association because of accusations of abuse of political dissidents and the adverse publicity of the appalling conditions of patients in the asylum of the Greek island of Leros. I gave several presentations at World Congree VIII, including presenting findings from the needs assessment study I had carried out in Leros with Jim Watson, Tom Craig, Paul Clifford, Yvonne Webb and Greek colleagues.[84] The situation at the Leros asylum was exposed by the *Observer* Sunday newspaper in September 1989; it attracted worldwide condemnation but also inspired compassion and a desire to help. Our involvement preceded this publicity, in an effort to assist in the reforms based on our experience with the

84 Bouras N, Webb Y, Clifford P, Papadatos Y & Zouni M (1992) A needs survey among patients in Leros asylum. *British Journal of Psychiatry* **161** (1) 75–79.

deinstitutionalisation programmes in our area of South East London. At the congress in Athens I also presented our model of community services for people with ID, in the presence of Frank Menolascino and Anton Dosen. Frank Menolascino had recently started the Section of Mental Retardation in the WPA and nominated as the next President Anton Dosen, who was very active in promoting international awareness of the mental health aspects of people with ID. I worked very closely with Anton Dosen and developed a strong professional and personal friendship, which has continued over the years to today. I contributed by establishing firmly the Section of Mental Retardation within the WPA structure.

At the Tenth World Congress in Madrid in 1996 the Section had a strong presence, with symposia and posters, which was assisted greatly by Professor Luis Salvador-Carulla and his Spanish colleagues as well as Mark Fleisher from Nebraska. Research outputs were gradually being produced from the study of mental health problems for people with ID and a variety of clinical reports on psychopathology were presented. In Madrid I took over the presidency of the Section and with the help of several colleagues, including Anton Dosen, Ken Day and Luis Salvador-Carulla, worked very hard to raise awareness of and interest in mental health problems for people with ID among general psychiatrists.

At the Eleventh WPA World Congress in Hamburg in 1999, in addition to several symposia and posters (which were all well attended), we launched the publication at the congress of a booklet entitled *ABC of Mental Health in Mental Retardation*, which was distributed to participants.[85] This publication offered basic knowledge on diagnosis, treatment methods and services for people

---

85 Bouras N, Holt G, Day K & Dosen A (eds) (1999) *Mental Health in Mental Retardation: The ABC for mental health, primary care and other professionals*. World Psychiatric Association.

with ID and mental health problems. It was received with amazing interest by the attendees and was highly praised by several colleagues, including Professor Ahmed Okasha, Chairman of the WPA Sections, as well as other members of the executive. Over the years, this booklet was translated into Spanish, Italian and Chinese, and was uploaded to various websites. We found this response of colleagues very rewarding, and we felt that we had started reaching the necessary critical mass of general psychiatrists to start looking at the issues related to the mental health problems of people with ID.

At the Twelfth WPA World Congress in Yokohama, Japan, in 2002, we attracted perhaps one of the best attendances at a WPA Congress in our Section's symposia and workshops. This time we had prepared a new publication on the basic aspects of autism and mental health, which was also distributed widely and very well received.[86] The presentations included more research studies on diagnostic methods, as well as studies on the effectiveness of pharmacotherapy and psychological intervention. Luis Salvador-Carulla took over the presidency of the Section in Yokohama. Professor Kosuke Yamazaki had invited Geraldine Holt and me to lecture in Tokyo after the congress. Geraldine talked about the development of our training and the programmes for supporting families and carers of people with ID and mental health problems, while I presented the issues related to services. That was a rather unique encounter, because when we arrived at the venue we found that we were in a proper theatre, full of people, staff, families and carers to listen to our talks – which were simultaneously translated into Japanese!

---

86 Holt G & Bouras N (eds) (2002) *Autism and Related Disorders: The basic handbook for mental health, primary care and other professionals*. London: Gaskell.

The Thirteenth WPA World Congress took place in
Cairo in 2005. There, Luis Salvador-Carulla, as president,
and Geraldine Holt, as honorary secretary, continued
the strong presence of the Section. This they also did
at the Fourteenth WPA World Congress in Prague in
2008, which was very well attended, and where Luis
Salvador-Carulla was also one of the keynote speakers.
Then Marco Bertelli took over as president of the Section.
He introduced the publication of a biannual newsletter
and prepared the programme for the Sixteenth WPA
World Congress in Buenos Aires, Argentina, in 2011,
where I was invited to chair the Section's symposium.
That was my last attendance at WPA World Congresses
and activities.

It was a very rewarding experience to grow from
a marginalised group in the late 1980s, to a strong
presence with worldwide recognition by general
psychiatry in the 2000s. The Section was strengthened
by the growing evidence-based research coming out from
different countries, as well as the activities of research
and clinically active centres on diagnostic methods,
classification systems, therapeutic intervention and
training methods. The Section was renamed Psychiatry of
Intellectual Disabilities, to be compatible in terminology
with other organisations. In addition to the above
mentioned activities, the Section participated in several
other scientific and training events, including joint
presentations with the European Association for Mental
Health in Mental Retardation/Intellectual Disabilities,
the European Psychiatric Association, NADD, IASSIDD
and others. The membership expanded in several
countries around the world. The Section also had a
strong presence at various WPA Regional Congresses
and related scientific and educational events.

In recent years, the Section was involved in a
working group with the WHO relating to the revision

of ICD-10 for the ICD-11, led by Luis Salvador-Carulla and Marco Bertelli. In this way, the Section made a major contribution to the debate around the classification of ID and documented the outcomes in published articles. I was invited to join an advisory group of colleagues, which I did with great interest, for this high-quality work was being carried out by younger colleagues.[87]

European Association for Mental Health in Intellectual Disability (EAMHID)

The success of the external training and other related events we organised with my colleagues at Guy's at the early stages of developing our services, together with the growing interest in community-based services, encouraged us to organise an international conference. It was the first time such an international conference had been organised in our field in the UK. With the help of colleagues from the Section of the Psychiatry of Mental Handicap of UMDS – David Brooks, Geraldine Holt, Katie Drummond, Sabah Sadik, Joanna Mulvey, Shaun Gravestock, Brendan McCormack and the administrator Pauline Formby – we booked the conference facilities of the University of Kent in Canterbury for 25-27 September 1991. The conference was also under the auspices of the Section of Mental Retardation of the WPA, whose president was Anton Dosen. In addition, we had invited on to the organising

---

87 In addition to colleagues mentioned above, others who collaborated with me during my time as president of the Section were Shoumitro Deb, Jane McCarthy, Henry Kwok, Gregorio Katz, James Harris, Michael Seidel, Jenny Torr, Giampaolo La Malfa, Karim Munir and others.

committee David Wilson from the Section of Mental Handicap of the Royal College of Psychiatrists.

The title of the conference was 'Mental Handicap and Mental Health: The way ahead'. The organisation was a mammoth task for us at that time and we had selected Canterbury as a pleasant but affordable residential venue that was close to London and easily accessible to overseas participants. The programme started on the afternoon of 25 September 1991, with keynote speakers Frank Menolascino, on 'International perspectives'; Steve Reiss, on the 'Assessment of behaviour and psychiatric disorders'; Ken Day, on the 'Specialised or generic services'; and Tony Holland on 'Down's syndrome and Alzheimer's disease'. There were six plenary sessions and six seminars, all delivered by invited speakers, who included most of the known colleagues in the field in the UK.[88] The conference received wide publicity and was attended by over 200 people from the UK and abroad. Geraldine Holt was interviewed about the conference on local radio, and the feedback was very positive. At the time, it was certainly a major scientific event for people with ID and mental health problems. Discussions and debates took place among so many internationally renowned colleagues, about almost every aspect related to mental health for people with intellectual disabilities. These discussions offered a momentum to accelerate collaborations and highly quality research and clinical activity for people with ID.

The success of this conference resulted in two

---

88 Yvonne Wiley, Bill Fraser, Sheila Hollins, Hillary Brown, John Corbett, Jeremy Turk, Vicky Turk, Chris Kiernan, Joan Bicknell, Shoumitro Deb, Jim Mansell, Jack Piachaud, John Clements, Lorna Wing, Greg O'Brien, Valery Sinason and Ann Craft. There were also several invited speakers from the US and other countries, including Betsy Benson, Andrew Levitas, Diane Cox-Lindenbaum, Paul Kymissis, Akihito Takahashi, Rangi Hagerman and Steve Weisblatt.

important developments. First, at the insistence of Frank Menolascino, I edited the book *Mental Health in Mental Retardation: Recent advances and practices*. Based mostly on presentations made at the conference, it was published by Cambridge University Press in 1994. Unfortunately, Frank did not live to see the book completed and it was dedicated to his memory. (I wrote his obituary for the UK daily newspaper, *The Independent*.[89]) The book was the first comprehensive text in the field and was reviewed favourably in the established psychiatric journals as well as those in ID. It was also included in the reading lists of several undergraduate and postgraduate courses. It is interesting that the most positive reviews came from the US, while reviewers in the UK wanted more evidence-based research, as there was not much evidence published at that time. Cambridge University Press published a second book following the same format five years later, and second and third editions were later published, all of which received excellent reviews.[90]

The second key development resulting from the Canterbury conference was the creation of the European Association for Mental Health in Mental Retardation – later renamed the European Association for Mental Health in Intellectual Disabilities (EAMHID). Anton Dosen was already active in the Netherlands organising

---

89 Bouras N (1992) Frank Menolascino: A pioneer psychiatrist in mental retardation (Obituary). *The Independent* **17** January.

90 Bouras N (ed.) (1999) *Psychiatric and Behavioural Disorders in Developmental Disabilities and Mental Retardation*. Cambridge: Cambridge University Press.
Bouras N & Holt G (eds) (2007) *Mental Health in Developmental and Intellectual Disabilities* (2nd edition). Cambridge University Press.
Hemmings C & Bouras N (eds) (2016) *Mental Health in Developmental and Intellectual Disabilities* (3rd edition). Cambridge University Press.

international events together with the training agency PAOS (Organisation for Post Academic Education in Social Studies). The first such conference was organised in Amsterdam in 1990. It was on 'The Treatment of Mental Illness and Behaviour Disorders in Mental Retardation', and laid the foundations for international collaboration at a time of growing awareness of the mental health problems for people with ID.

With the expansion of the European Union, the need to start a European Association focused on the mental health issues for people with ID was discussed in a series of meetings between me, Anton Dosen and Ken Day.[91] It was at that meeting that the creation of the European Association for Mental Health in Mental Retardation was agreed.[92] The main aims of the newly formed European Association were to improve mental health care for people with ID, which it sought to do by organising scientific meetings, exchanging expertise, stimulating research and promoting continuing professional development courses. In addition, the European Association aimed to offer advice and support to organisations and governments on policy and practical matters related to mental health for people with ID.

The membership was opened to organisations and individuals from psychiatry, psychology, medicine, pedagogy, nursing, social work. I drafted the constitution of the association for approval at the first annual general meeting (AGM), which was planned to

---

91 Anton called a meeting in Veldhoven, Netherlands, in October 1992, which was attended by colleagues from Netherlands, UK, Italy, Belgium, Greece, Germany, Spain, Denmark, Croatia, Switzerland and Sweden. Robert Fletcher and Louis Fusaro attended as representatives of the NADD.

92 The first members of the executive committee were Anton Dosen (Netherlands), Ken Day (UK), Willem Verhoeven (Netherlands), Christian Gaedt and Wolfgang Meins (Germany), Marcel Van Walleghem (Belgium) and myself (UK).

take place at the first European Congress in Amsterdam on 13-16 September 1995. This congress was very successful, and was attended by over 500 people from 24 countries (including the US, Australia and Japan). (The membership of the European Association included colleagues from 13 countries.) The programme included round-table discussions and symposia covering diagnostic issues, psychotherapy and pedagogical approaches, together with workshops, free presentations and posters.

Among the new topics that emerged from this congress were genetic defects and their link to psychiatric and behavioural disorders, systems approaches to psychiatric problems, cultural aspects relating to the care of people with mental health problems and ID, and organisational aspects of care. An additional feature of the congress was the introduction of pre-congress courses. The European Association organised eleven such courses, covering subjects including inpatient systems therapy, psychiatric and behavioural aspects of fragile X syndrome, diagnostic approaches in behavioural and psychiatric disorders, counselling and psychotherapy, pharmacotherapy, and the multidisciplinary team approach to severe behaviour problems. Together with David Brooks and Theresa Joyce, I delivered a course on the training package we had developed for staff supporting people with mental health needs and ID. It was a very successful congress and the feedback was very good.

At the end of the last century, the Second European Congress, on Mental Health in Mental Retardation: Services, training, and research for people with developmental and learning disabilities, provided an excellent opportunity to learn from experience gained over the years and to examine new research findings. The congress was organised in London by the European Association for Mental Health and Mental Retardation, in collaboration with the Royal College of Psychiatrists' Faculty of Learning Disabilities, the NADD, the WPA Section of Mental Retardation, and the IASSIDD SIRG-MH.

The congress took place in September 1999 at Brunel University, in Uxbridge, Greater London. The Estia Centre, with several colleagues, were were heavily involved with the organisation of the congress. The expectations were high and the organisation of such events had by now become quite sophisticated, involving also serious financial risks. The administrative infrastructure of the European Association was relying mostly on voluntary input from a small number of people. We chose Brunel University conference facilities for the same reasons as we had chosen the University of Kent in Canterbury for the International Conference in 1991. The choice of Brunel instead of the University of Kent this time, was in order to be closer to London and hence more convenient for the overseas participants. This time we contracted CATS to run the Congress; however, CATS was unfortunately declared bankrupt the year before the Congress was to take place, causing us a major headache. Fortunately, Pavilion Publishing stepped in and undertook the organisation of the congress, but the transfer of organisation from CATS to Pavilion Publishing was not without problems that required extra time and attention before solutions could be found.

Over 400 delegates from 24 countries attended the congress. Topics ranged from ethical issues to service provision, from biological research to treatment options, from specific disorders to challenging behaviour. The choice of parallel sessions, seminars and workshops was extensive. Many of the speakers were internationally known and almost every colleague known nationally in the field of mental health and ID was present.

At end of the congress there was a debate, sponsored

by the Faculty for the Psychiatry of Learning Disability of the Royal College of Psychiatrists, and discussing the statement, 'There is no place for mental health legislation for people with intellectual disabilities'. The debate was chaired by Oliver Russell, proposed by Tony Holland and opposed by Greg O'Brien.[93] We received very good feedback and the success of this congress established the presence of the European Association as an important organisation promoting quality education, training and R&D in the field.

The Third European Congress, Mental Health in Mental Retardation: Theory and practice, took place in Berlin in September 2001. This time it was organised by the German Society for Mental Health for People with Mental Retardation on behalf of the European Association. The organisation was led by Michael Seidel and aimed to provide an international platform of experts to present scientific results, points of view, important ideas and questions on prevention, diagnosis, treatment, service provisions, training and research aspects for people with mental retardation, developmental and learning disabilities, and mental health needs. There was again a very rich programme over three days, featuring keynote speakers, seminars, workshops and so on. More research and evidence-based practice was emerging across several countries, and this congress provided the opportunity for some groundbreaking debates and discussions. This time, the host organisers also put together a very interesting social

---

93 The following were elected members of the new Executive Committee at the Second European Congress: Anton Dosen (Netherlands), president; Nick Bouras (UK), vice president; Geraldine Holt (UK), secretary; John Hillery (Ireland), second secretary; A van Gennep (Netherlands), treasurer; and members Giorgio Albertini (Italy), Pat Frankish (UK), Carina Gustafsson (Sweden), Neil Ross (France), Luis Salvador-Carulla (Spain), H. Seppala (Finland), Michael Seidel (Germany), Willim Verhoeven (Netherlands), Germain Weber (Austria).

programme, which gave us the opportunity to explore Berlin.

The publication of the new European Association *Practice Guidelines for the Assessment and Diagnosis of Mental Health Problems in Adults with Intellectual Disability* was marked at the Berlin congress.[94] This publication was led by Professor Shoumitro Deb, who was well known nationally and internationally. The publication , was very well received and attracted a lot of interest, not only from the participants at the congress but beyond, and it is still in circulation. The book was reviewed favourably in different professional journals and was translated into Dutch and Spanish. It is not an exaggeration to state that this publication, as well as those by the Section of the WPA referred to above, have become 'classics' in their field.

The Fourth European Congress, 'Mental Health in Mental Retardation: A lifetime multidisciplinary approach', was held in Rome in September 2003. This time other organisations contributed to the organisation of the congress, namely, the Italian Society for the Study of Mental Retardation (SIRM), IASSIDD, the Section of Mental Retardation of the WPA, NADD and the International Society on Early Intervention (ISEI). Giorgio Albertini of Fondazione San Raffaele led the organisation of the congress, together with Marco Bertelli, Giampaolo La Malfa and Alessandro Castellani from SIRM. The venue was the Domus Mariae in the historic Via Aurelia in Rome. Giorgio Albertini was an excellent organiser who had hosted several international meetings in Rome before this congress, as part of the Ageing Round Tables of IASSIDD. The programme was even richer than the previous congresses; there was increased participation

94 Deb S, Matthews T, Holt G & Bouras N (2001) *Practice Guidelines for Assessment and Diagnosis of Mental Health Problems in Adults with Intellectual Disability*. Brighton: Pavilion Publishing and Media.

from all over the world and contributions advancing the evidence base of mental health matters in people with ID.

I was invited to deliver a keynote speech on 'Service developments for persons with mental health needs and ID'. Anton Dosen talked on 'Progress in assessment, diagnosis and treatment of psychiatric and behaviour disorders among persons with ID', and Michael Seidel presented on 'Human rights, participation and mental health'. The continuation of the publication of the Mental Health Special Issues of the JIDR and the biannual publication of the European Association newsletter had been given a new impetus. Michael Seidel took over the presidency of the European Association at that time, and Marco Bertelli (Italy), Giampaolo La Malfa (Italy), Nigel Beail (UK), Patty van Belle-Kusse (Netherlands) and Ramón Novell Alsina (Spain) joined the executive as new members. Over 500 people attended this congress who at the end endorsed the 'Declaration of Rome' (presented to them by the congress organisers), which called for 'promoting, facilitating and extending opportunities of real participation for people with ID in all professional activities'. Concern was expressed about the continuing neglect of the mental health needs of people with ID in several European countries, and the participants, as part of the declaration, also called for 'the politicians in all European countries to meet the demands of mental health provision and the development of necessary support for people with ID and additional mental health problems'.

The Fifth European Congress, 'Mental Health in Mental Retardation: Integrating research and practice', took place in Sitges, Barcelona, in October 2005. This time the congress was organised in collaboration with the Spanish Association for Scientific Study on Mental Retardation, Sant Joan de Déu Mental Health

Services, under the auspices of the Health Department and Social Welfare and Family Affairs Department of the Government of Catalonia. The organisation of the congress was led by Ramón Novell Alsina, together with Luis Salvador-Carulla and José Garcia Ibañez. The success of this congress was beyond any expectation. The programme included keynote speeches, and a great variety of seminars and workshops on almost all topics related to mental health and ID. Several pre-congress courses also took place, and all were very well attended.

After this congress I left the executive of the European Association, which I had served since its inception. I left having spent many hours organising several events, but also with the satisfaction of knowing that my personal contribution had helped to create international interest in improving the quality of life of people with mental health problems and ID, through R&D and training. The next congress of the European Association was held in Zagreb in 2007 and the European Association that has continued to thrive to this day. Subsequent congresses were held in in Amsterdam in 2009, in Manchester in 2011, in Estoril, Lisbon, in 2013, and in Florence in 2015. The European Association was certainly one of the main vehicles for promoting awareness in mental health problems for people with ID; and MHiLD and the Estia Centre were among the important contributors.

In 2017 the 11th Congress of the European Association of Mental Health in Intellectual Disability will be held in Luxembourg. I have been invited by Professor Germain Weber, Chairman of the Organising Committee, to deliver the keynote speech, in which I will share my reflections from my long-standing career and contemplated the future.

Journal of Intellectual Disability Research, Mental Health Special Issue

The activities of the European Association were attracting increased interest, so in 1995 we decided it was time to publish a new journal focused on mental health and intellectual disabilities. We were very keen to include NADD in this venture and I started discussions with Robert Fletcher, with whom I had raised this possibility as far back as 1993. At the same time, I approached Blackwell to explore the possibility of publishing the proposed new journal. I had many exchanges of ideas with Robert Fletcher, who though interested in the idea was reluctant to commit NADD to publishing a new journal based in the UK. Blackwell was also undecided about the publication of a new journal at a time when there were radical changes taking place in the journals market thanks to the introduction of the internet and the significance of the impact factor.

Then Bill Fraser, who was the editor of the *Journal of Intellectual Disability Research* (JIDR), a well-established journal in the broad area of intellectual disabilities, came up with the idea of the JIDR becoming bi-monthly instead of quarterly, and for one or two issues to be assigned as 'Mental Health Special Issues'. I became the first editor of the Mental Health Special Issue of the JIDR, and the inaugural issue was published in 1996, in association with the European Association. Over the next decade, we published 20 special issues, and these were very well received. I believe that the publication of the Mental Health Special Issues contributed significantly to raising the profile of mental health related issues for people with ID, and stimulated research and evidence-based practice. In the meantime, Bill Fraser retired as editor of the JIDR and invited me to apply to succeed him. He was persuasive, and I applied with some reluctance. I regretted my decision, though I was disappointed because I was not appointed. Instead Tony Holland was appointed as editor of the JIDR, and we worked amicably together for the rest of my time as editor of the Mental Health Special Issues, until my retirement.

NADD decided to publish their own official journal in 2008, entitled the *Journal of Mental Health Research in Intellectual Disabilities*. I was honoured to be invited by Robert Fletcher to become the editor, but I declined, insisting that as the journal was US-based the editor should be too. I accepted the position of consulting editor and worked together with Johannes Rojahn, the first editor of the *Journal of Mental Health Research in Intellectual Disabilities* who was succeeded by Angela Hassiotis. A year earlier, in 2007, the Estia Centre had published *Advances in Mental Health in Learning Disabilities*, as an evidence-based practice journal (see Chapter 10). This was it's own entity and not in competition with the research-oriented journals, JIDR's Mental Health Special Issues and the *Journal of Mental Health Research in Intellectual Disabilities*.

More international activities

It should be noted that in addition to the international activities described above, I and my colleagues from MHiLD and the Estia Centre had been involved in a plethora of other training, teaching, research and development activities. These included some long-standing collaborations on research and development projects; organising workshops; and lecturing at local, national and international events. Among these activities was the long-standing collaboration with Anton Dosen in the Netherlands, and Luis Salvador-Carulla, Ramón Novell Alsina, José Garcia Ibañez and their colleagues, who were mostly in Catalonia but also in other parts of Spain, including Cadiz and Cordoba.

The collaboration with Luis Salvador-Carulla started in 1991 during the congress in Canterbury. Then he had visited me in my office at Guy's to ask advice about developing mental health services for people with ID in Spain. Thus began a long-lasting collaboration and warm friendship that continues today. I also acknowledge the innovations in Spanish services that were led by Dr Juan Pérez Marín, president of one of the main NGOs that provided care for people with ID in Spain, particularly in Andalusia. Strong collaboration was developed with Italian colleagues Giampaolo La Malfa, Marco Bertelli and Alessandro Castellani, who on several occasions invited me and my colleagues to different parts of Italy to lecture or meet service officials and administrators. John Hillery was also a regular collaborator in Ireland, together with Nicola Wolfe, who worked as a CPN in our service, and her husband Joe. Visits to Ireland were always very fruitful and enjoyable. Henry Kwok, who was trained by us at Guy's was also a regular collaborator in Hong Kong and organised training events there. For several years there was also ongoing collaboration with Nancy Cain and Philip Davidson of the Strong Centre in Rochester, New York State; Jenny Torr, Bob Davis and Bruce Tonge of Monash University in Melbourne, Australia; as well as with Chad Bennett of the University of Melbourne, and Nick Lennox and Nikki Edwards in Queensland. Bruce Tonge and I worked together during my first job in Britain at St John's Hospital in Stone, Aylesbury. Joint publications produced with most of our collaborators have documented our joint working. I also maintained a regular strong cooperation with colleagues in Greece, including Professor Takis Sakelaropoulos, a pioneer of community mental health in Greece since the 1980s; Professor John Tsiantis, a strong advocate for community child mental health services and reformer of the Leros asylum (and with whom I worked on European Union funded projects); Professor Costas Soldatos, an initiator of several innovative training and research activities; George Christodoulou, member of the WPA executive, John Tsegos, creator of the Open Psychotherapy Centre in Athens; Costas Stefanis, ex-president of the WPA; and Dr Tasoula Karastergiou and her colleagues in Thessaloniki, who were also pioneers of psychiatric reforms in Northern Greece.

All of the international work mentioned in this chapter was most important in offering me an insight into and first-hand knowledge of the trends of psychiatry around the world and, most importantly, on developing services. It was also of great importance for personal development, not only for me but for my colleagues with whom I have worked closely over so many years.

Several countries have progressed into the post-institutional era, while for others community care still remains an ambition to be fulfilled. The issues and dilemmas of what constitutes the most appropriate services for people with ID and mental health problems have been addressed by different countries and become the focus of important policy initiatives in recent years. The strong international collaborations of MHiLD and the Estia Centre have offered a facilitating platform for these developments on training, capacity-building and research.

Epilogue

The Project Group that started in 1982 with the aim of improving the quality of people and service users with ID who were in long-stay institutions, eventually enlarged to cover catchment areas serving over one million inhabitants in four London boroughs, and developed an academic centre. Throughout all of these years, feedback and participation from service users, their families and carers was strongly encouraged and has always been at the centre of all actions.

The Project Group took a team approach with many participants; this lead to success and satisfaction, but also problems and disappointment.[95] I feel perhaps we, with colleagues at MHiLD, should have tried harder to be more persuasive and influence policy on the mental health needs of people with ID. None of the problems, however, overshadow the great role of the NHS in the provision and delivery of a wide range of mental health services in the UK. Having seen several other systems around the world, through the international work described in this book, I believe that the NHS is a unique system, offering universal access for the whole population at the point of contact.

I retired from my clinical and academic positions in 2008 after having worked at Guy's Hospital for 35 years. I was greatly honoured to attend the

---

95 Bouras N & Holt G (2010) *Mental Health Services for Adults with Intellectual Disability: Strategies and solutions*. Hove: Psychology Press.

Festschrift Conference organised by my colleagues at Guy's Hospital and held on 16 January 2008. Tribute presentations were given by psychiatrist my colleagues Graham Thornicroft, Shoumitro Deb, Jean O'Hara, Colin Hemmings, Jed Boardman, Tom Craig, Dimitrios Paschos, Geraldine Holt, and Jim Watson gave a personal tribute. Lynette Kennedy spoke from nursing, Alison Little from Southwark Social Services, and Stuart Bell, Phil Woods and Mark Allen from the management. Peter Tyrer read a poem, which is still framed in my office.

I handed over my role as clinical director to Jean O'Hara, the R&D to Jane McCarthy and the training to Steve Hardy. A year later, in 2009, there was another great honour for me, when Graham Thornicroft and Jean O'Hara unveiled my portrait, painted by David Cobley, at the HSPR Department of the David Goldberg Centre.

Following my retirement in 2008, Graham Thornicroft hosted me in the HSPRD and entrusted me, together with Stuart Bell, CEO of SLaM, and Professor Peter McGuffin, then Dean of the IoP, with the development of Maudsley International. Maudsley International is a major joint initiative of the Institute of Psychiatry – now the Institute of Psychiatry, Psychology and Neuroscience – and South London and Maudsley NHS Foundation Trust, that promotes training, teaching, research, service developments and consultancy worldwide in the field of mental health. The aims of Maudsley International are to improve global mental health by sharing expertise with colleagues from all over the world. Maudsley International was founded on the principle of integrating academic and clinical interests, and at its heart is the translation of expertise from research and training into high quality practice on the ground. Maudsley International are providing access to a wide range of expertise, through programmes that combine clinical, academic, managerial, policy and intervention knowledge to inform developments in other places. Maudsley International offers services tailored to the needs of colleagues working in very different environments around the world. It does this by providing unparalleled opportunities to share best practice in clinical and professional practice, governance and performance management, quality and productivity, knowledge transfer through training and development programmes, change management and leadership, strategy and policy development and implementation, service models and service systems. These activities, for example, include service reviews and evaluation, mental health promotion and well-being, social inclusion and recovery, user empowerment and rights and ethics. Maudsley International has become a community interest company under the Maudsley Charity and has been involved with programmes in over 40 countries around the World. Tracey Power, who first worked with me on the closure of Grove Park Hospital (see Chapter 5), is the managing director of Maudsley International, supported by me as programme director; Jonathan Rolf as director of business, strategy and operations; and a board, with Graham Thornicroft as chairman, and Norman Sartorius, past president of the WPA, and Paul Farmer of Mind as non-executive directors.

In 2011 I was invited to coordinate the Research Advisory Group of the Daedalus Trust. The Daedalus Trust was funded by the three founding trustees: Lord Owen, Lord Chandos and Lord Skidelsky. The objectives of the Daedalus Trust are the advancement of education for the public benefit, by conducting research (and publishing the useful results of that research) into the personality changes associated with the exercise of power among leaders in all walks of life and its effect on decision-making. The combination of risk-taking tempered by wisdom, as demonstrated by the Greek mythical character Daedalus, suggested the name for the trust and its projects. It indicates the negative consequences of behavioural risk management. The ancient Greek concept of 'hubris', or arrogant pride, was considered to be one of the most dangerous traits one could exhibit. According to the classical Greek myth, when Minos the King of Crete refused to surrender a beautiful white Cretan bull for sacrifice, Poseidon demanded that as punishment, Minos' wife, Pasiphae, would fall in love and adulterously mate with the bull. A son was born, the legendary Minotaur, with the head of a bull and body of a man. In response, the shamed Minos demanded that Daedalus, the renowned architect, construct a labyrinth to hide the Minotaur. Later Minos blamed Daedalus as an accomplice in the killing of the Minotaur by Theseus, and Minos imprisoned Daedalus together with his son Icarus. Daedalus and Icarus, trapped in the labyrinth, sought to escape by flight. Daedalus constructed wings for himself and Icarus and warned his son to keep a middle course, in order to avoid being too close to either the moisture of the sea or the heat of the sun, as he had used thread and wax to make the wings. At first, all went well, but eventually an overly exuberant Icarus flew too close to the sun. The wax wings melted and he hurtled downwards into the sea. Icarus' hubris, his disobedience of his father in flying too high, is a cautionary tale about humility and restraint, the sin of presumption.

In modern times, hubris refers to the negative consequences of actions that appear to be associated with arrogant decision-making based on a lack of knowledge or interest in and exploration of facts, combined with overconfidence and a lack of humility. The Daedalus project seeks to encourage the interdisciplinary study of the concept of individual and collective hubris, and the possible effects on personality of exposure to power and the isolation and veneration that often accompany it.

Since my retirement I have also been actively involved in the activities of the Section of Psychiatry of the Royal Society of Medicine, where I have been supporting my colleague and friend George Ikkos in the development and delivery of an innovative and successful programme of lectures, entitled Psychiatry in Dialogue with Society.

This book is a personal account of reflections from my professional and life experience of 35 years in British psychiatry. I witnessed major ideological and system reforms, as well as spectacular research and technological discoveries and innovations. I have tried to present here a personal view of what it felt like, having worked for so many years as a psychiatrist at the front line of the clinical, academic and mental health management worlds. I have been very privileged to be included in a work environment that embraced respect and encouraged novelty. The needs of service users have always been at the centre of efforts to ameliorate their suffering and improve their quality of life.

In 2011, over 30 years since the start of the resettlement of people with ID, an unfortunate incident of neglect, the Winterbourne View abuse scandal, led NHS England to accept that more than 2,000 people with ID and mostly mental health and challenging behaviour problems were placed in hospital-type facilities.[96] Since then, a new wave of policy documents has been released – some of them very prescriptive – on how to reduce the numbers of people with ID being kept in hospitals, mostly in the private sector,

---

96 Transforming Care and Commissioning Steering Group (2014) *Winterbourne View – Time for Change* [online]. Available at: https://www.acevo.org.uk/news/winterbourne-view.

for unnecessarily long periods.[97,98,99,100] From the Green
Light Toolkit (see Chapter 10), to Blue Light and
Fast Track!, it is astonishing that the reasons for the
regrettable phenomenon of placing people with ID in
hospitals, even today, are not explicitly recognised. In
this book, the failure over time to properly develop the
necessary specialist services has been well described.
For example, the use of CPA is emphasised in recent
policies, though it has been shown in previous chapters
of this book that there was resistance to the application
of CPA (see also Chapter 10). Though the policy makers
are well-meaning in their intentions to create the
right environment and structures for a better quality
of life for people with ID, it is nevertheless surprising
that they do not take into account the implementation
evidence of previous policies before introducing new
ones. Ideology, together with lack of knowledge and
expertise, are among the main problems; financial
constraints are not the only factor.

The clinical practice of psychiatry cannot be
viewed in isolation from trends in society and culture.
Deinstitutionalisation, community care, normalisation
theory principles, advocacy, empowerment and recovery
are some of the main products of strong sociological and
ideological views that prevailed in psychiatric practice
during my time. These ideologies have had more impact
on the care of patients with severe mental illness

97 NHS England (2015) *Building the Right Support* [online].
    Available at: https://www.england.nhs.uk/wp-content/
    uploads/2015/10/ld-nat-imp-plan-oct15.pdf.

98 http://www.england.nhs.uk/wp-content/uploads/2014/11/
    transformingcommissioning-services.pdf

99 NHS England (n.d.) *Transforming Care* [online]. Available at:
    https://www.england.nhs.uk/ourwork/qual-clin-lead/ld/transform-
    care/.

100 NHS England (2015) *Care and Treatment Review: Policy and
    guidance* [online]. Available at: https://www.england.nhs.uk/wp-
    content/uploads/2015/10/ctr-policy-guid.pdf.

Reflections on the Challenges of Psychiatry in the UK and Beyond

and intellectual disabilities than molecular genetics and neurobiological research. I also worked through major reforms in service systems and practices. I had the opportunity to experience the two systems of the NHS and the university, which complimented each other in medicine, including psychiatry, through the appointment of what were known as 'clinical academics'. This meant consultants acting as clinicians, but also fulfilling academic duties in teaching, training and research. Today the separation of the two systems has deprived psychiatry from the twofold contribution both in clinical practice and research and development.

The current dominance of neurobiological research perspectives notwithstanding, psychiatrists need to have a deeper understanding not only of brain function, but of social factors, the environment, relationships and culture. Psychiatric disorders are aetiologically complex and their origins cannot be explained in simple terms. At times, psychoanalysis, early biological psychiatry, social psychiatry and, most recently, molecular psychiatry were strongly advocated for psychiatric disorders. Explanatory pluralism is preferable to monistic explanatory approaches, especially biological reductionism. Psychiatry must embrace complexity and support empirically rigorous explanatory and pluralistic explanatory models.

A conceptual reorientation in how we think about mental health care is a necessity. In today's complex landscape of services for people with mental health problems, the number of possible interfaces between services is increasing. Together with existing uneven financing systems, these interfaces are increasingly difficult to manage in terms of providing personalised care pathways that are adjusted to the needs of service users and their carers and families. A new concept of 'meta community mental health care' is more suitable for the current status of mental health services. This is the topic of an article I have been working on with my colleagues George Ikkos and Tom Craig. The principles of post-community mental health services should consider mental health as a public health issue and should conclude that both physical and mental illnesses are real, complex biopsychosocial phenomena, requiring a pluralistic approach to mental illness, understanding and treatment, parity of esteem, and equity of access to physical and mental health. The aim should be compatible with the vision of the United Nations 2030 Agenda for Sustainable Development, adopted by the General Assembly in September 2015, that strives for 'a world with equitable and universal access to quality education at all levels, to health care and social protection, where physical mental and social well-being are assured', and where 'all human beings can fulfil their potential in dignity and equality and in a healthy environment'.[101]

---

101 United Nations (2015) *Transforming Our World: The 2030 agenda for sustainable development* [online]. Available at: https://sustainabledevelopment.un.org/post2015/transformingourworld/publication.

Abbreviations

AHMT: Adult Health Mental Handicap Team
AMH: Adult Mental Health
ASD: Autistic Spectrum Disorders
ATC: Adult Training Centre

BDU: Behavioural Disorders Unit
BILD: British Institute of Learning Disabilities

CAG: Clinical Academic Group
CAMHS: Children and Adolescent Mental Health Service
CAT: Cognitive Analytical Therapy
CIT: Crisis Intervention Team
CMHT: Community Mental Handicap Team
CPA: Care Programme Approach
CPN: Community Psychiatric Nurse
CQC: Care Quality Commission

DH: Department of Health
DHSS: Department of Health and Social Security
DPP: Diploma of Psychiatric Practice

ENCOR: Eastern Nebraska Community Office of Retardation
ECR: Extra Contractual Referral

FTs: Foundation Trusts

IASSIDD: International Association for the Scientific Study of Intellectual and Developmental Disabilities
ID: Intellectual Disabilities
IoP: Institute of Psychiatry
IoPPN: Institute of Psychiatry, Psychology and Neuroscience

GP: General Practitioner

JIDR: Journal of Intellectual Disability Research

KCL: King's College London
LD: Learning Disabilities
LSL: Lambeth, Southwark and Lewisham Health Commission

MHAC: Mental Health Advice Centre
MHiLD: Mental Health in Learning Disabilities
MIETS: Mental Impairment Evaluation and Treatment Service

NADD: National Association for the Dually Diagnosed – renamed National Association for Developmental Disabilities
NHS: National Health Service
NGO: Non-governmental organisation
NICE: National Institute of Health and Clinical Excellence
NIMHE: National Institute for Mental Health in England
NSF–MH: National Service Framework for Mental Health
NUPRD: National Unit for Psychiatric Research and Development

PAS-ADD: Psychiatric Assessment Schedules for Adults with Developmental Disabilities
PASS: Programme Analysis of Service Systems
PCG: Primary care group
PCT: Primary Care Trust
PICU: Psychiatric Intensive Care Unit
PIN: Planning for Individual Needs

R&D: Research and Development
RAE: Research Assessment Exercise
RCT: Randomised Controlled Trial

SELHA: South East London Health Authority
SETRHA: South East Thames Region Health Authority
SHA: Strategic Health Authority
SIRG-MH: Special Interest Research Group – Mental Health
SLaM: South London and Maudsley

UCLA: University of California, Los Angeles
UCSF: University of California, San Francisco
UMDS: United Medical and Dental Schools (Guy's and St Thomas' Hospitals)

WPA: World Psychiatric Association

Other titles from Nick Bouras, The Estia Centre and Pavilion Publishing

Mental Health in Learning Disabilities: A training resource

by Geraldine Holt, Steve Hardy and Nick Bouras
This comprehensive training pack introduces those who support people with learning disabilities to a range of important areas of knowledge and practice, from understanding mental health and psychiatric disorders, assessment of mental health problems, challenging behaviour, epilepsy and autism, to different types of interventions, legal and ethical issues, service factors, cultural diversity and offending behaviour. Each module provides all the material needed to run a short training session within the context of a staff meeting or training event. Includes a copy of the new supporting handbook Mental Health in Intellectual Disabilities.
Available from: https://www.pavpub.com/mental-health-in-learning-disabilities/

Mental Health in Intellectual Disabilities: A reader – Fourth edition

by Nick Bouras Steve Hardy and Geraldine Holt
In recent years there have been many changes in the field of mental health and in services for people with intellectual disabilities. With this in mind, this fourth edition of the reader has been completely revised. Two chapters are dedicated to the new legal and policy frameworks that are now in place and include information on the Care Programme Approach (1990), the revised Mental Health Act (2007) and the Mental

Capacity Act (2005). There are also chapters on specific mental health problems, which offer greater insight into how carers can recognise such problems, and how they are diagnosed and treated. Supporting people with personality disorders and those who misuse substances is an emerging issue for services and is also examined in this edition.

Available from: https://www.pavpub.com/mental-health-in-intellectual-disabilities/

Supporting the Physical Health Needs of People with Learning Disabilities: A handbook for professionals, support staff and families

by Steve Hardy, Eddie Chaplin and Peter Woodward
As well as looking at the challenges of accessing healthcare and navigating care pathways, this handbook presents a practical guide to the most common conditions and health needs, with chapters written by experts in those conditions and their relationship to learning disabilities. A range of issues are covered, including mental health, cancer, epilepsy, respiratory and swallowing problems, and poor sight and hearing.

The book aims to increase awareness and knowledge of how these conditions and issues present themselves, as well as how they can be prevented in the - rst place and best practice inassessment and treatment. It will therefore be a valuable resource for families, support workers and health professionals.

Available at: https://www.pavpub.com/supporting-physical-health-needs-of-people-with-learning-disabilities/

An Introduction to Supporting the Mental Health of People with Intellectual Disabilities: A guide for professionals, support staff and families

by Steve Hardy, Eddie Chaplin and Karina Marshall-Tate
People with intellectual disabilities are more likely to experience mental ill-health than the wider population for a number of reasons including biological, social and psychological vulnerabilities.

This introductory guide uses common language in order to demystify mental health and illness in the lives of people with intellectual disability. The varied content contains a number of case studies illustrating common mental health problems, and explains how people with intellectual disabilities can be supported to protect their mental well-being.

It provides guidance on treating a person with intellectual disability for a mental health problem, adaptations to treatment that may have to be made, and how best to find the right services for an individual with intellectual disabilities and mental health problems. Available from: https://www.pavpub.com/an-introduction-to-supporting-the-mental-health-of-people-with-intellectual-disabilities/

The Mini PAS-ADD Interview Handbook: 3rd Edition
by Steve Moss
The PAS-ADD system is a family of assessments that has gained worldwide recognition for its contribution to improving the mental health assessment of people with intellectual disability (ID). Although the initial impetus for developing the system was for the particular needs of people with ID, the PAS-ADD assessments are equally valid for the general population. They are particularly valuable in situations where the person has more limited language skills. They are also excellent for

use in research projects demanding high quality data on symptoms.

The Mini PAS-ADD was initially developed in recognition of the fact that many health and social service professionals have detailed knowledge of the client, but may not have a formal background in psychiatry or psychology. The Mini PAS-ADD provides a clinical glossary that includes examples of each symptom at various levels of severity. This glossary enables highly reliable estimates of symptoms to be made. The interview also has questions to guide the interviewer in asking about the symptoms.

Newly revised and fully updated to be compliant with both ICD-10 and DSM-5, the Mini PAS-ADD covers a range of common mental health problems. There are sections on anxiety, depression, bipolar disorder, obsessive-compulsive disorder, and psychosis, as well as a screen for autism spectrum disorder. In addition, the Mini PAS-ADD includes a small constellation of symptoms that were identified in the original field trials as indicating the presence of an organic disorder.

In the 15 years between the development of the 1st version and this 3rd edition, the Mini PAS-ADD has become widely used around the world and has been translated into a variety of languages. During this period, the author trained several thousand people in the use of the PAS-ADD system, and the experience gained through this has led to the development of this current edition.

Available at: https://www.pavpub.com/the-mini-pas-add-handbook/

PAS-ADD Clinical Interview handbook

by Steve Moss with Robin Friedlander
The PAS-ADD Clinical Interview has been designed to

meet the particular problems of assessment in people with intellectual disabilities, but is equally valid for use with the general population. It provides full diagnoses under both the ICD-10 and DSM-IV (TR), and also provides a framework for producing a wider case formulation using other assessment frameworks (behavioural, ecological, psychodynamic etc).

The interview is designed to maximise the possibility of conducting a clinical interview, even if the client's level of language is poor. Questions are also provided for informants so that the interviews can be conducted with a client and informant, or just with an informant if the client is non-verbal. Information can be collected not just on current mental state, but also on a second representative episode.

The PAS-ADD Clinical Interview uses a scoring system that is transparent to the user, making it very clear to see not just the criteria that have been fulfilled but also those that are close to fulfilment. This makes the process of clinical interpretation easier and based on clear evidence.

Available from: https://www.pavpub.com/pas-add-clinical-interview/

Challenging Behaviour and People with Learning Disabilities: A handbook
by Steve Hardy and Theresa Joyce

This handbook is an essential resource for those working with or caring for people with learning disabilities and behaviour that challenges. It provides timely and essential guidance to ensure that there is a competent workforce that can provide effective, ethical and high-quality support.

People with learning disabilities who have behaviour that is describes as challenging are one of the most vulnerable groups in society. They are at risk of being excluded from services, being denied opportunities and being placed away from their local communities and families. They are also more vulnerable to poor practise and abuse.

This user friendly and accessible resource emphasises the importance of respecting people who use services, their families and carers.
Available from: https://www.pavpub.com/challenging-behaviour-a-handbook/

The Mental Capacity Act and People with Learning Disabilities: A training pack to develop good practice in assessing capacity and making best interests decisions
by Steve Hardy and Theresa Joyce
This training pack introduces the Mental Capacity Act, its principles and associated issues to all staff working with people with learning disabilities. It covers defining and assessing capacity, making best interest decisions and Deprivation of Liberty Safeguards. The content of this pack will develop the skills and knowledge of staff in using the act in practice. It aims to empower people with learning disabilities to make their own decisions and ensure the rights of those who lack capacity are upheld.
Available at: https://www.pavpub.com/the-mental-capacity-act-and-people-with-learning-disabilities/

Guided Self-help for People with Intellectual Disabilities and Anxiety and Depression
by Eddie Chaplin, Jane McCarthy, Steve Hardy, Lisa Underwood, Debbie Spain, Peter Cronin, Liam Peyton and Jayne Henry
Guided Self-help for People with Intellectual Disabilities and Anxiety and Depression is a multi-media training resource developed specifically for

people with intellectual disabilities. It compromises a printed manual with guidance for facilitators who are supporting an individual to use the self-help resource (SAINT), as well as a Self-Assessment and INTervention resource that uses colour photographs and easy read text to deliver structured and accessible guided self-help with this population.

Available at: https://www.pavpub.com/guided-self-help/

Autism Spectrum Conditions: A guide

by Eddie Chaplin, Steve Hardy and Lisa Underwood. Published in association with the Estia Centre, this guide provides a comprehensive introduction to working with people who have autism spectrum conditions (ASC). The book addresses the needs of people with ASC across the lifespan and across the range of intellectual functioning. Though the content is grounded in evidence-based practice and recent research, the text is intended to be as practical as possible, offering insight into the everyday lives of people with ASC and how staff can best support them.

This guide is for staff working in health and social care services, as well as families, carers and anyone else who supports people with autism spectrum conditions, with or without additional learning disabilities.

Available from: https://www.pavpub.com/autism-spectrum-conditions/

Mental Health Promotion for People with Learning Disabilities: Supporting people with learning disabilities to stay mentally well

by Steve Hardy, Peter Woodward, Sarah Halls and Ben Creet

This training pack is for learning disability professionals and others who wish to facilitate a course to help people with learning disabilities improve their mental health by raising awareness of mental health problems and developing personal strategies to improve or maintain their mental health. The 12-session course is designed to be run with adults who are able to express their wants and needs and who need minimal support with daily living tasks.

Based on work with The Tuesday Group who have spoken and published articles about their work in this field, the pack includes a wealth of mental health promotion materials, including video role plays, and is structured into 2 ½ hour interactive sessions. https://www.pavpub.com/mental-health-promotion-for-people-with-learning-disabilities/

Working with People with Learning Disabilities and Offending Behaviour: A handbook
edited by Eddie Chaplin, Jayne Jenry and Steve Hardy
This handbook is designed to provide the reader with information on forensic issues in people with learning disabilities. Covering the same topics as the training resource, it reflects the latest developments in services and treatment for this group. The handbook can be read independently or used to support the training course materials contained in the accompanying training pack.

Professionals within the social care sector are required to undertake Continuous Professional Development (CPD) by the General Social Care Council (GSCC) and those who use this resource will be able to gain CPD points.
Available at: https://www.pavpub.com/working-with-people-with-learning-disabilities-and-offending-behaviour-handbook/

Working with People with Learning Disabilities and Offending Behaviour: A training resource
edited by Eddie Chaplin, Jayne Jenry and Steve Hardy

This training resource offers a range of professionals an introduction and framework to the issues, legislation and practice around working with people with learning disabilities and offending behaviour.

Written by a range of contributors from multidisciplinary backgrounds, this accessible resource provides invaluable background information and learning opportunities for all those working in forensic services for people with learning disabilities. The training material is organised into 12 modules, each supported by a chapter in the companion handbook. The training can be provided as stand-alone modules or as a comprehensive course, and is designed to be delivered by trainers and/or clinicians who have experience in providing forensic services to people with learning disabilities.

Available at: https://www.pavpub.com/working-with-people-with-learning-disabilities-and-offending-behaviour-training-resource/

Index

Organisations are listed by full name:
see p.215-17 for acronyms.

Reflections on the Challenges of Psychiatry in the UK and Beyond
© Pavilion Publishing and Media Ltd and its licensors 2017.

Reflections on the Challenges of Psychiatry in the UK and Beyond
© Pavilion Publishing and Media Ltd and its licensors 2017.